In The Footsteps Of A Bipolar Life

Life Writing

Abigail George,
Ambrose Cato George

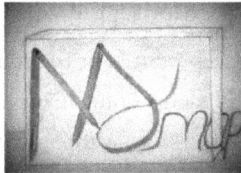

Mwanaka Media and Publishing Pvt Ltd,
Chitungwiza, Zimbabwe

*

Creativity, Wisdom, and Beauty

Publisher: *Mmap*

Mwanaka Media and Publishing Pvt Ltd

24 Svosve Road, Zengeza 1

Chitungwiza, Zimbabwe

mwanaka@yahoo.com

mwanaka13@gmail.com

https://www.mmapublishing.org

www.africanbookscollective.com/publishers/mwanaka-media-and-publishing

https://facebook.com/MwanakaMediaAndPublishing/

Distributed in and outside N. America by African Books Collective

orders@africanbookscollective.com

www.africanbookscollective.com

ISBN: 978-1-77933-137-3

EAN: 9781779331373

DISCLAIMER

All views expressed in this publication are those of the author and do not necessarily reflect the views of *Mmap*.

Foreword

My dad is one of the lucky ones. His voice merges alongside mine like beautiful scraps of material. This is a story about a man but not about any man. It is a story about my father. Fathers are special people. Mostly they encourage you. You tell them about your list of goals and in return, they inspire you to fulfil them. They are the ones standing on the sidelines. They are the ones who give you that standing ovation. They are the ones who mouth the words 'I love you' and 'I think that you are brilliant' when you feel like you did not do as brilliant as you should have. They are the first ones you go to when you feel sad or when you are happy. All my life that is what my father did. He was not all of those things all of the time. Sometimes he was sad and as a child, it made me feel very angry and confused when daddy cried or was upset. Now, I imagine him as a young adult as a hunter. A lonely warrior whose head was bursting out of his skull, his brain cells tormented by the Periodic Table, smashed up against elegant words like bilateral symmetry, biology, anatomy, dissect, zoology and mitochondria surrounded by a mountain of books, hills and green valleys of physics and chemistry textbooks. My father was like a beautiful shadow, my beautiful shadow that always lingered in my presence. We will talk for hours on everything and nothing at the same time. I do think that I am a poet because of him because are not all writers are poets at some stage in their lives or at least have the potential to become poets within them. He is a writer and a teacher who wanted to become a medical doctor but life had other plans for him. He has been writing all his life to get to this point in time and even now, he is always in pursuit of something or other. He believes in many things and most of all his spirituality, the nature of his soul is like that constellation beyond the trees. Primitive, ancestral, universal and that of a dream catcher. My father is a funny and sweet man. Understanding

3

my love for this funny and sweet man who in his own words has had a curious relationship with his hair on different continents and with the pencil test, whose life story reads like a book of secrets, claustrophobia, vertigo, therapy and it has set my life journey on a trajectory that is (simply put) out of my hands. Human beings do not know as children whether they are truly destined for great things. Whether or not they will be the follower or the leader but all children have the potential for greatness. What unlocked my dad's greatness? I really do not have an answer for that question. Maybe that surprises you. Maybe you expected me to say that perhaps it was his depression or the fact that he had a mental illness. Most of all, I want your life to be changed by this man's life and the people who came to love him when he was at the crossroads of the depths of despair, isolation and rejection (and don't we all fear rejection) and the edge of hypomania. I think that every person who suffers from a mental illness has a hidden life. When you are depressed, it is another habitat. You are closed off from the rest of the world. Shut off from the rest of normal (what is normal anyway) humanity. You are in that void, that black hole separated from the people who love you the most and there is nothing, nothing that can bring you back from that brink. People tend to think that people who suffer from a mental illness cannot recover completely from it (I think people who think like this think that recovery is the furthest thing from their mind). Depression damages people and that is a fact. The ego has a mind of its mind here when it comes to chronic illness and the road to recovery. I have seen my funny, sweet, generous and forgiving father happy and unhappy. Seen lucky him, my best friend, through laughter, tears, and the grim winter of depression.

25 October 2015
Abigail George

Chapter 1
A Beautiful Mind

I, Abigail George am at Hunterscraig. I am here because I am not coping anymore. I am not coping because I am not the doctor. Because I am not the pharmacist with their jagged little pills. With their pharmaceuticals. Because I am not the one who is fluent in the doctor's language no matter how hard I try. How will I be able to benefit from wearing that white laboratory coat, stethoscope around the neck, with that particular bedside manner? Where is my infinite piano? Watch this. Watch this romance. It is clever math, no; it is elegant math with all of its violent alertness under my fingertips. What is the weather like in Los Angeles? What is a winter like in Los Angeles? What will my head say to my heart as I walk on that beach, or breathe in that valid air from that Parisian meadow with my moral compass to navigate me on those open roads, the wide open spaces of the Midwest? What will my limbs say to each other in London if I ever get around to having that London experience forgoing all my responsibilities as a writer and a poet in South Africa? For isn't that what I am first and foremost. A South African writer and poet living in a post-apartheid apocalyptic city. City life as opposed to life in the rural countryside. Searching for greener pastures in the asphalt garden where everything is golden and chameleon-like. I have never wanted the experience of loss. The measure of loss but life has given me that responsibility. Sutures too. And panic and I have had to thread both against threadbare knuckles. I have covered myself up with an American quilt. It has become my shroud. It has become my cover in other poetry. But I feel it all the time now. The warmth of anxiety. I feel it humming, humming, and humming in my bones. Singing to the leaves on the winter trees. Guests every one. They're like bees. They're a rapturous swarm. What do I know without having a sophisticated culture, a knowledge and education beyond this tidal moon and sun and then I think of the planets. How like the planets I am? I know my place. I know my place so well now that I cannot give it up. And why would I? There will never be a case of mistaken identity. All I will ever know about life is the predictions of Sappho, poetry and writing. And how sometimes how beautifully unpredictable life can be otherwise. There are storms in the dark and we need to speak about the acute pain from those storms in beautiful and wonderful ways. Mostly the image of depression is that of a wild thing. When I'm crazy I know that is when I am most alive. When I am not crazy, when I am most sober is also when I am most alive but I don't know it. All feeling leaves me and I long for the stress of crazy. I long for someone to tell me I'm beautiful. And to the mock wife that I would give my eternal screaming life for. You are mine. The pain of Sarajevo is in my blood. Mingled there in my blood. Staring back at me in my blood and but what can I do but stare back at it? The door was somehow left ajar for me and my heart was bursting. It ready to be split open like a pomegranate. Seeds everywhere like seawater. I found wild oblivion, the safe passage from suffering in those seeds. At first I could not speak of the fantasy that I held in my hands and that my head wished for so ardently. I could not interpret those promised lands that my mocking husband returned from. I needed land and yet I needed to be reborn as well. I needed stress, a tour of the flesh like I needed the back of my hand. I flickered and then I was buried once again amongst the flowers. And with dirt upon my head I soon realised that I was supposed to be the beautiful keeper of the vanished and the unexamined. The apprehended. I do not want to age. To age means to give up your mortality like an artist giving up their brushes. To age means to give up everything. To age means that you are not bold anymore and that you don't have anything to be brave over. It just happens to be in your blood to think these things. Never mind how you try not to. I need to write to you of the quiet courage of our mothers and our grandmothers. So pay attention to my birthday notes. Grief is only a warning. Denial too. I need to find out why the brightness dies so effortlessly and with artful commitment. The heart of commitment. And the flowers heads. Every one. The night is blue. The night is dying and whatever flame of light and love I have treasured in my hands from the smiles of my children with bars of chocolate in their hands those are the walls of my prison cell. Inside my head there are brick walls. In my arms there are cells too like the laughter of clowns. The pathetic frustration and laughter of clowns that will never be enough. Nobody deserved this. Nobody deserves this depression and the lid of this pressure that catapults them from yesterday, today and tomorrow.

I, older, wiser, with a family of my own now find myself at the local swimming pool. The air is cool. The temperature is freezing as I pull the sweater over my head. My limbs have found freedom in a sense. My children have already found themselves in the water. I can hear them laughing. It makes my heart smile. I leave the stressors of the daily grind behind me. I long to pull away from the wall and to kick my legs as if I was swimming in my childhood quarry again with my friends. I can feel my heart hammering inside my chest. In the water my limbs find a harmony. I find a harmony. This is something precious. A father spending time with his children. My oldest has a faraway look in her eyes. She has just started high school and every pang, every hurt that she feels I feel it too. The other two are just babies. They know nothing of the grown up world and I thank God for that. That they will remain children and innocents for a while longer. I wish this with my whole heart but already I feel that I have damaged them irrevocably in some way. I wish I could turn back the past but I can't. It is out of my hands now. I do not know what will happen in the near future. I know nothing of my failure as a parent to protect them from the dangerous and shark infested waters of this cruel world. I know nothing yet of their own failures.

They're so innocent. I look upon the magnificent angelic shine on their faces. Those were the days I worshiped the ground their mother walked upon. I climb down the steps at the side of the swimming pool. I feel as if I am an authentic unique. The water gets a hold of my legs. It takes a few minutes for me to gather my bearings. I feel the weight of water around me. My older daughter's face is sullen. She has not become rebellious yet but I know that one of these fine days she will refuse to pray with us. She will give me the silent treatment and the cold shoulder as the chip that she carries on her shoulder grows and grows. She will no longer be the loving dutiful daughter she once was and tell me all her secrets. She will no longer think of herself as being beautiful and wonderful. She will begin to see herself as less than perfect, less than extraordinary, less than beautiful and wonderful. She will, and it breaks my heart to say this, begin to see herself as flawed. Her mother will become less familiar to her because she will find it therapeutic to spend quality time with her other children who see no wrong in her. And then she stretches out her arms and begins to swim elegant stroke after elegant stroke. She loses herself in the womb ceremony of the water. She finds herself here.

My wife and I have never discussed having prodigies for children but prodigies they are but aren't all mother's children prodigies? I have been an educationalist for decades now so I am the expert. I know what I am talking about. I have met many gifted children who have had no one sadly to believe in them and so they have been lost through the system and the establishment. These gifted children have had no platform and so they have in return become delinquent and criminal. The girls have become shop assistants and lovers and the young men work at menial labour toughening themselves against the injustices of the world that they find themselves in. They get married too early. They have those kids too early and sometimes they become fathers when they are mere children themselves. Their sunny road is not sunny for long and so they turn to alcoholism and the insanity of addiction and sometimes become demagogues yielding violence and brutalising their wives, their children and their families. I have met all of them in my teaching career and I saved those that I could save. I saved those that were in my power to save but unfortunately I could not save every one when their parents themselves are lost too. There were times when I came too late on the scene, on the scenario.

Madness is a hands down bloodied affair. Madness is much more than searching with your whole heart for sobriety from addiction. This time around my stay at Hunterscraig was a few weeks. I sat and listened to my children my muscles tired, aching and sore. Afterwards we would get cool drinks for everyone. Sometimes ice lollies, popsicles, sweets, caramel popcorn and bubble gum. Things that children would enjoy. I would get the morning paper if I had not read it yet at school with my morning tea and sandwiches. Under water the images I had of other people, other people and my children's reality would appear blurred, unnatural and disturbing. They would all appear surreal, Dadaist, subliminal. The love a father has for his children will make him weak at the knees. It will make him realise his own limitations, his own flaws and his own weaknesses. I will always remember the touch of my first love, that first empty page, those clean lines of that notebook that I filled with scrawl scribbling away, my dogs, my children's birthday parties, the wards at Hunterscraig. High care, the discreet nature of madness. How ordinary madness could be, how cool it was for the James Deans of the world but not for you and the wuthering heights of it. I thought of Bethlehem a lot. Don't ask me why. Maybe it was because of the illness, the nature of it. I try not to think of the most disturbing things that I felt and that I saw and that of course happened to me. The sodomy. The rape of a young man. A man who was younger than me and clearly out of his sane mind. He did not realise what was happening around him. I did not try and encourage myself to remember anything when I left the hospital or that posh clinic. I wanted to leave it all behind me. I wanted to embrace the life I had with my wife and three children. I had worked hard for it. I had sweat blood and tears for it. I needed to do the right thing by my wife. She had stood by me so now it was all up to me to stand by her. Rituals are intensely felt especially religious rituals.

And when I want to calm the anxiety that rises again and again like sweet waves with those jagged little pharmaceuticals this is how I remember Helen Martins. The Magi and the Owl House; their tethers tug like flame at my heartstrings and I wonder about her wounds, her coy magical healing, did she ever prepare a delicious, warm cake for her friend, that social worker that Fugard spoke so highly of. What stalked her for so long; a lifetime and then she had to go and die still so young, fighting fit? Oh, suicide is a forlorn, lonely way to go. Don't do it, I would have said and she would have looked at me. Our eyes, I imagined would have connected the way the white sunlight connects with the angles and corners of shadows of furniture, against the wall, against the panes, against panels and cupboards, on summertime afternoons and then I would have understood her motives, the intention behind it all, the mystery, the spell that 'it', suicide, had cast over her, her life's work and as I wander through her house I can feel her presence. Her perfect presence. She was that most perfect thing. She was that most perfect artist. I don't think her unstable. She doesn't haunt me, my waking thoughts as much as her body of magnificent work, her 'art' does; if I can call it that. Writers write, poets lose themselves in translation, philosophers who pose as academics during the day intellectualise debate over wine and sushi until the early hours of the morning. When did she know her jig was up, that her time had come to bid this cruel world adieu in the worst possible way? Who found her with her insides eaten away? I read Fugard's The Road to Mecca. I was jealous. Jealousy and cowardice are in the sticky blood of every writer and it simply does not boil away to a faint, hot zone of grieving nothingness, fumbling bits and pieces like crushed autumn leaves dead in the centre of the flushed palm of your hand. Helen's Mecca cast its own spell on me. To me it felt magical. A love spell launched into the language of the pathways of a warring fraction of nerves, anxious to please like a child with the limbs, eyes, soft, sweet-smelling tufts of hair and a smile of a doll's features and yet, a spell that was blank up front, to take comfort in that blankness as if it was purified like a chalice of Communion wine and it was also a spell that spelled, 'be faithful as a servant of God, a man of the cloth'. So what if I am not the Doctor. So what if I am not the pharmacist. I am in a ward of crazy thirsting for sobriety. He, Fugard, seemed to craft the impossible in a way that did justice to Helen, the insecure, little, belittled bird afraid of the outside world; Helen, the Outsider in a way I knew I could never because I did not get the 'hook', the 'bait' but fishing for information, our keen sense, our powers of observation of human behaviour is what writers and poets know best as we drink our coffee, brew pots of tea, grow a hunched back bent over our ancient computer. How did she, Helen who was not so insecure after all, build that wall around her? How did she approach each subject, each project; as an assignment? Did she miss the feeling of the warmth in her bedroom of another human being? The company of her dead husband, their daily rituals filled with breakfasts, hot, buttered toasts, meals that came out of cans, processed foods that could easily be heated up and eaten with bread like pilchards or sardines. They would probably have imbibed hot drinks during the day; warm milk at bedtime, lukewarm tea when it was called for, the bitter taste of coffee with grounds at the bottom of the cup in the morning. I think she had an inkling she would live on even in death and in her gift that she left to the world, was the method in her madness. Colour Me In. Colour in those apparitions. Did these apparitions that came to life see her as a mystic; a prophetess bound for crucifixion and resurrection, with her own shroud of Turin, God forbid, did they come to life under her splayed fingertips, come to her from above, heaven-sent, as natural as night and day? Were they angelic utterances whispered in her ear while she slumbered, as she turned in her sleep, twisting the sheets between her legs until finally she dreamed until daybreak or were they the of hallucinations induced by the isolated landscape, the barren countryside which surrounded her, the wilderness of her antisocial behaviour of her own making, induced by the mind of a woman slowly going mad, losing common sense, lacking that quintessential backbone of what made the English, the liberal-minded, so organised in their group or sporting activities like tennis for example, cricket or high tea; activities that required teams and cliques, so formal even in their games, proud of their progeny that followed in their footsteps, productive in the world, a world of their own making that was to a certain extent selfish, self-absorbed, not welcoming and friendly to people they considered to be not a fit partner in their climate; so genteel were they and conservative in their broad outlook on life. When I read of how people take their lives into their own hands I wonder what will happen, if there will ever be any substantial record of proof of their life here on earth. In the end, does it really matter to them, I question, yes, perhaps I judge their actions harshly and too quickly but to me it does matter because I was brought up that way; to believe that there is something holy and godlike about your spirit, your soul, your physical and emotional body and to take what does not belong wholeheartedly to you is stealing and there is nothing pretty about being caught after the act. If only, I imagine people who stumble across, infiltrate the place where the deceased lays, the body arranged in death, find the fragile creature as if taking a nap, resting, face composed, still, nothing amiss except the silence in the room where the unfortunate act of defiance, of quiet desperation had taken place without anyone's knowledge. You learn and you live to surrender. You learn to let go of the past and live. If only, I had come sooner, not said this, said that in a moment when all my thoughts were focussed perfectly, perhaps if I had acted swiftly but depression is both mean-spirited and long-suffering and there is no escape from that if it is passed down from generation to generation, inherent in the highly feminine woman prone to emotional outbursts, hysterics, tantrums, panic attacks, melancholy, mania, self-medication with painkillers and potions brewed with herbs and the effeminate man. Most people live in altered states of minds when something traumatic has happened to them. Most people think that therapy can help them with this. Sitting down face-to-face with someone who has studied the maladies of the mind for years and years they bare the deepest, darkest secrets of their soul and then leave, feeling relieved, as if they have just done something noble. They think they will find the answers their soul is seeking once a week ongoing sometimes for several years or for their natural life. They find someone who they feel is suitable, someone motherly, fatherly or someone young who reminds them of a loved one, someone they lost or who even reminds them of their own children or a substitute for the absent parent from their childhood and adolescence and young adult life. But I was really writing this about Helen Martins and for her, in defence of her and of the life she lived. Some people just can't help making waves and the more flawed they are, the more they can't stop making waves. Perhaps she found the answers she was looking for, the elegant solutions she craved like scientists or mathematicians craved in their own work, in her art, her sculptures, her friendship. I wanted to make sense of her thinking. What was it, inside her head that was making her tick insatiably, behind her eyes that was making her see, what exactly was her fruitful, the blooming flowers of her subconscious telling her to do, willing her to do consciously, conscientiously, consistently, efficiently and at a time unbeknownst to the world at large while she was still alive. In death, she has survived it all that she couldn't in life and yet she is still remembered as a woman made of skin and bone; a bone-woman, shapeless, caught in a thoroughfare like kittens to be drowned in a bag; her features like a sandscape, opening and shutting, through which seawater spills. Martyrs are made of this. And whenever I am troubled my thoughts turn to Gethsemane and whatever was deathly illumined there. I lived in a brutalised society when I was a child. I witnessed my mother and my father arguing back and forth sometimes, back and forth relentlessly. I think of my own violent alertness when it came to anything cultural, knowledgeable and educational. It is both an explosion and a stagnation. The church. This dream world at large that is both poetry-flecked. How my golden flesh and the notebook from my heart that rhythm vibrates and resonates and I want to say to God. The living God that I worship and can find no wrong with. I want to say to this angelic host that he is my earth, my stone and rain and that he is most of all is my Sappho. He is the frame of my spirit. And of course all the tenderness of the natural world. Madness is just another sickness that will make you tremble. That will make you weep Remember this. That there will never be anything extraordinary about that. I don't need to love or be loved in return As much as I need to swim towards the light. Towards the illusion that is both honesty and hostility keeping the dog on the leash as he discovers the minutia in the essences of humanity. Children playing in the child's world in childhood dirt. The gardener planting, soil erosion, the fields, the roses and the altered states of mind that keeps humanity under wraps. For is not the church not another country? Far and away beautiful and lovely. A bride holding a book. The pages majestic. The pages smelling of roses. And together we will discover why humanity is important to humanity? Why is poetry needed? By poets and humanity alike? And night I make tea or my daughter and we escape to the sitting room. I wonder at the bittersweet oranges we use to make holes in when we were children and suck the juice out of them. Why skin and hair? The tapestry of flesh. I need trees and leaves Grass and the seasons. Precious mountains and wild life with all their simple orchestrated movements. The unmistaken frame and rapture of it all. There's beauty in everything in the simple ceremony of pouring tea. Drinking it primitively. The sunrise is in the image of a woman. Her femininity. What would we call that muscle? Would we call those wings lungs? A well of tidiness. Springing up relentlessly. There's blood in the old life. Blood in the new one. Prospering breath after breath. So empires are built. The crown of laughter Poetry and studying the poem's death underneath the surface of it all. Whatever is in the nature of praying meditatively and of discovering happiness behind the aloof façade of illness and mental sickness? Sickening creative ritual and impulse is where I live now. I live yonder. I could not choose words. Because I did not have it within me to possess me. I only had everything that glistened. When will this impulse end? I did not call for it. I did not want to possess it. Although I know now that it wanted to possess me infinitely. The only response that I had was to shed tears, was for my physical body to be wracked with sobs and with every sob and with every story a light would shine on this illness. I needed hysteria. I don't know why. I just know this. That I needed it. And then I found a leap of faith. The beginnings of a leap of faith. And I turned towards the face of God. I found honour and privilege there. And in the whine of language I found something else. Writing soothed my soul like nothing else did. Writing calmed the storms with black clouds that still had those patterns of silver linings within my heart. Hysteria is fashionable. Do you know how fashionable it is? Grief is fashionable too. Grief for your old life and your old ways of thinking. I am still here. I am a father and a grandfather. I am no longer a son. I have to fight. I have to fight this mental sickness. And that is why I have to fight because I am loved and because I love and because I am surrounded by the face of love. Illness will never dwindle in my life. It will always have its own turning point. It will always have its own pawns and revolutionaries. I know I need to make adjustments to my character and my personality. To cope, to live, to rejoice jubilantly that after all of this with my heroic friends that have passed on to the hereafter, my friends who have crossed over that I am still here. It is night time. It is night land in this posh clinic at the end of the world. I of course only think that it is at the end of the world. I cannot fall sleep. I have been here for weeks now. My children are put to bed at night by my wife. I cannot know of course what she is thinking, feeling and dreaming. I only know that perhaps she carries all the burdens of the world on her shoulders tonight. I love her. God knows how I love her. But I don't quite know how she loves me. She does not know yet how to let go of me. She does not yet know how to surrender me to the fabric of time and the tapestry of the universe. I do. I do. I do. But we have taken vows in a church in front of our family and all of our friends. All of those unified lethal elements. It is cold. It is a winter's night. I drink a glass of water and wonder what it is made of. I think of the Periodic Table. Teaching it to a classroom filled with misfits who have no idea of their own genius and potential. Once upon a time before I was a principal of a school I was an inexperienced chain-smoking manic depressive teacher. I didn't think then that I had it in me to be a principal of a school. I didn't think I had it in me to be a leader but I became one in the end and was it because of everything I experienced or in spite of those challenges. In spite of those obstacles that turned out to be opportunities in disguise throughout everything. I don't know.

In flashbacks and dreams I am at Elizabeth Donkin or I am at Valkenburg. Ingrid Jonker's Valkenburg a scholar of trivia clutching my packet of smokes and pharmaceuticals.

Chapter 2
For a Youth in the Northern Areas

I miss my mother more and more every day. But on our wedding day she was my Cinderella. I was her prince. For the young making love is just for fun. I have never read Charles Bukowski, William Faulkner, D.H. Lawrence, Nadine Gordimer, and J.M. Coetzee. I've never even heard of Salinger. They have all swept my eldest daughter away. Sometimes I think to myself will she ever be a bride? Will she ever fall in love? Feel what her dad felt as he looked at his new wife. With our married life ahead of us. A day old. Will a man ever take her in his arms and say, 'I love you best?' But these are just the thoughts of an old man in the autumn of his years. This morning I felt depressed. The world can do that to you when you're infirm. You think nothing will ever hurt you again. You're built like an impenetrable fortress in the mountains at the end of the world. Our marriage had promised us new beginnings. Wonderful beginnings. But now there's silence. I cry for what I have lost. Not real tears. Just a sob or two that wracks my body. She's not so far away from me. The two double beds are in the same room. Gerda is reading by the light from a lamp while I search for my pharmaceuticals. Swallow my tablets as if they were aspirin. Curbing my enthusiasm as I watch her disrobe. Looking at her now I realise how much I still love her. Let me count the ways. Love has a delicate smell. It means to offer you the rituals of sacrifice, buying a house, moving furniture, a wife by the name of Gerda staring at her reflection in the mirror while she brushes the tangles out of her hair, pats her hair down, puts a stocking on and wraps a scarf around her head. She is still beautiful, but not just to me, to other people as well. I still think I didn't deserve her. Is she happy? Have I made her happy? She stayed with me for better or for the worst. I ministered to my children. I lectured my children when it needed to be done. To set them straight. To set them on their life journey. Their pilgrimage of sorts. And I took them all, my loving, boisterous family from hell to an eternity of hell. And of course in the wards of hell, or the wards of Valkenburg, there is not much of a presence of becoming indoctrinated by religion. I didn't find Buddha when I was in Valkenburg. I didn't turn in a Brahmin. I was only introduced to that much later when my children were teen-agers. Things like meditation. I did give up smoking, but not red meat. Wiping the fat off my lips. I never drank much. I hated the stuff. I saw what it did to my own father. Gerda is silent. In her own world, and I wonder (it is not for the first time) what is she thinking about? Does she still love me as much as I love her? What I wouldn't do to embrace her like I did the first night of our married life? I hate this loneliness that is flowering inside of me like a lotus. I must write about what I like, what I mesmerises my all-knowing, all-seeing eyes, about the difficulties of married life, the first meal my wife cooked for me as my wife, how I watched the movements of my wife at our wedding feast set out in a church hall, filled with Johannesburg people, and a few members of my family. I must write about what makes me emotional (yes, even men get emotional, over-excited about the annihilation of evil by good). I must write about what makes me misty-eyed, what cuts me deep where the depths of suicidal illness awaits, watching my children in Victoria Park playing while I watched them from afar, sitting on a park bench that was once reserved for Whites only in a White people's park. Over weekends the park would usually be deserted. I'd get chocolate and packets of crisps for the children. I'd see their smiles. Their laughter and sticky fingers would lift me. Give me a buoyant mood. Perhaps you are sensing that I am not telling you the whole truth. There were days when I had to force myself to get out of bed. I was a man who had plenty of responsibilities. I couldn't just give in, quit life, quit family life, lie on the sofa, stop taking cold, refreshing showers that restored some vitality, some energy to my brain, and clarity of thought, vision and self-actualisation to my insight. I couldn't escape my children, I couldn't not acknowledge them (their pain was my pain, their emotional fabric in time, was my emotional fabric in time and place, and their moments of childhood depression stopped me dead in my tracks). I couldn't just quit my children's world, divorce their mother, live without the difficulties of a husband, live in a bachelor pad with relative freedom, no domestic responsibilities from their world, because they needed me. My family needed me. And as I watched my small children looking at all the things I couldn't buy for them (their choices they already knew had to fit my pocket), things like that would melt my heart in the Greek's shop, and as they carefully made their purchases I was eternally grateful that I had made it through another day. I had made it through another manic depressive episode. No more aspirin for me. I had put Valkenburg behind me. There was Elizabeth Donkin, and the beginning of lithium therapy. There was my beautiful wearing blue jeans, a comfortable jersey that I had seen her in many times, and a white shirt. There was my wife getting out of the car. I was waiting for her on the steps of ward F. Waiting for her perfunctory kiss on the cheek. Waiting to sit down in well-worn chairs.

'How are you?'

'I've missed you.'

'I've missed you too. When are you coming home?'

Well, the conversation would go something like that.

I watched her shield her eyes, looking, looking, and looking for me. And then her field of vision changed. Her eyes met mine. And then she was locking the car door. Making her way towards me with that day's newspaper, a selection of magazines, bottles of juices, or a fruit basket. And the depression, with its elated highs that felt so invincible, that made me feel exquisite frustration, the faith that I had that the feelings were killing me, every day would come with their turning points. My heart was suicidal depression's apprentice. My brain was its master. I put my wife on a pedestal, but did she know it? In the beginning before I was married, I thought of all women as sex objects. Did I tell her how much I loved her? I worshiped the ground she walked on. Before her I was not romantic. Before I met my future wife my style and technique of a lover was dry when I was depressed. She made me into the man I am today. Throughout it all she convinced me to choose life, discriminate death. For every season there is a senseless tragedy. In love nothing is insignificant.

'Off to the old age home with you.' She said the other day. It broke my heart to hear her say that. We don't make love anymore. We sleep in separate beds. There's a distance between us now that I can't describe. It has no time or place. It's like a bridge. If we stayed together or even for as long as we have it is only because of the children. Sometimes I wonder what my wife was like as a child. The grief she must have felt as a young child after losing a sibling, a brother. But we never spoke about things like that. I never yearned to ask my fiancé, or new bride anything that would make her feel uncomfortable. In her eyes, I wanted to be give her only good memories. I wanted to make her forget about the pain of her childhood the way she made me forget about my own painful childhood. How I was bullied, terrorised on the playground, teased, called names.

As a child I was a watcher, a dreamer. I was always in love with books. With self-learning. With teaching myself new things about the world around me. Life experience. That's what White people called it. White people had cars. White people sold. White people were business minded professionals. When I was a child I fell in love with education. Maybe that's when I became a teacher. In childhood. I had an unquiet mind. I still do. There are a lot of rituals when I go to church on Sunday morning. There's the breaking of bread and Holy Communion. It's not real wine of course. It's just grape juice. I'm a changed man when I leave the church (less depressed. I feel less lonely. I don't know why that is. Maybe is has to with the biochemistry of the brain, or social activities, being involved in something even if it is as mundane as going to church). And the bread is not the thin wafers we used to get at the Union Congregational Church that the children looked at so longingly in their innocent hearts with that angelic shine on their faces. My wife and I would bite into the wafers. With that one bite the body of Christ was now part of our spirit, our soul consciousness, our physical bodies. Abigail couldn't understand that she had to be confirmed before she could partake of the body of Christ and the drinking of grape juice. She told me that we (it was always we even though I was the one behind the steering wheel of the car) road past Mrs Turner in the street, and that although Mrs Turner (Abigail called her Mrs Turnip behind her back after that day) saw us, must have recognised our car she didn't wave back. Well her body is all weirdly shaped like a turnip was Abigail's thought and I told her that's what happened to people as they got older. Everything physical changed and sometimes they started to forget things too like their manners (etiquette to Abigail).

I just smiled and then I laughed and said, 'Really? Maybe she didn't see us.'

'Daddy, really? Are you sure? She looked right at me and I waved and I waved and I waved and she still didn't wave back.'

I couldn't tell her this then. She was too young. An innocent. They could hurt me, but I would not let them hurt my children.

The following year we started going to Pearson Congregational Church which was situated in Central. Everyone who went there was White. You love your children. You really do whether they've done something good or bad. You're the one person in the world they can to when they need anything. If they ask you for money you bend down and you tell them to pick the money off the money tree. You tell them that you love them because that is the remedy for everything. When they're sick you nurse them back to health. When it's their birthday you buy them a cake, presents wrapped in brightly coloured paper, blow up balloons, and you give them a party and invite all the neighbourhood. You give them a hug when they it the most even when they're at their most rebellious nature. Shower them with fatherly concern when giving advice. It's also your honour, and privilege to provide daily inspiration from a verse in the Bible, to school projects. But when they get depressed of course you worry for them. You have discussions behind a closed bedroom door in the middle of the night that go and go on until the early hours of the morning and you think back to when you were in high school. I was from a different generation. The more things change the more they stay the same. Isn't that what the adage says? Should we all go and talk to someone like a family counsellor, a therapist. Gerda was always the one who was two steps ahead of me. She didn't come out and say it or tell me what she was thinking. She took Abigail when she was barely out of her teens to a psychiatrist who studied in Vienna. He had wild hair like Einstein. She had been prepared for an eventuality of this magnitude. She was the one who had been prepared. Not me. And there was a part of me that felt like a failure. I had been completely blindsided. I had not seen the diagnosis coming. Not from a mile away. My beautiful, darling daughter. My darling, darling daughter was a manic depressive just like me. Bipolar. Bipolar. Bipolar. I was struck dumb. Speechless. What could I say? How could I comfort her? She hated school. She hated every minute every second of it. A monumental waste of her time it was she said. She already knew that everything she was being taught came out of a textbook that supported the cause of a colonial master. That supported a White cause. A liberal's issues. Not hers by a long shot. We had to do a lot of talking, and listening, and the having of more conversations behind a closed bedroom door at night to try and convince her to stay in school. They were lots of tears. Everybody cried. There were arguments. There were times when she stayed with her aunt in Johannesburg and we would be under the false impression that now everything would be all right again in her world. We had dreams for me. She was brought up with norms and values. And we didn't, couldn't just let her throw her life away like that. Somehow, somewhere when she was fifteen years old she had written away to The London Film School. 'So she wants to run away to London now.' Gerda sighed. She wore a perplexed look on her face, chewing her bottom lip in pensive mode. I thought back to Abigail's last words of the conversation the three of us had, mother, father, with their rebellious, fiercely intelligent, highly temperamental daughter. 'I hate you.' She almost spat. 'You're killing me. If I stay here I'll die. You'll see. I'll show all of you. I'll kill myself if I don't go to film school. I want to go to London.'

Gerda had more intuition, knowledge and insight into how females thought and bonded and suddenly at midnight she bloomed. Her face pale in the moonlight, with aquiline features that her daughter Abigail had inherited from her but not her tennis legs or her mother's love for that game. I couldn't make out her face but I knew it was shining full of love for me, and for our daughter. All three of our children had been conceived in love.

'Where will she stay? Where will she sleep? What will she eat every day for breakfast, lunch, and supper? Is she sleeping now I wonder? She just sits glued in front of that television all hours of the day and night. Ambrose tell me, what do you think I should do? We? Us? She'll never be accepted. I read that story. It's terrible. But if I say that to her it will break her heart. She's fifteen going on sixteen.'

Back and forth my flashbacks goes. Presently we are here. The house is quiet haunted by ghosts from the past. Stephen. Jean. Magdalene. My parents. Gerda's own mother and father passed away when Abigail was still a baby. Baby Ethan is sleeping soundly between his parents on their double bed. He is a real busybody. He only has eyes for his mother. Already he has two milk teeth which has everyone in a frenzy in the household.

I wish sometimes that I had listened more, praised her cooking skills (even though she burnt the pots more times than I could keep track of), given more attention to my wife. Had not treated her like I had treated all the women in my life. Indentured slave girls only there to make me tea, be my secretary, flirt with. Women who would stroke my ego given the chance. She had given me everything of herself that she could as a wife, but I had not been completely open with her. Only in retrospect when I look back at the events of the past decade and they shaped all three of our children's futures did I see how selfish and arrogant I had been. I had not come clean. Pharmaceuticals cannot wash away sins. With my silence I had passed down three life sentences. I wish I had done something. Said anything to console my wife it would be twenty years until we got our daughter back. Have I made Gerda happy, and what about my children, are they happy? Are they successful? Have my children fulfilled all their childhood goals? People change from one generation to the next. That's the thing with people, milestones and events. They are always changing, and yet always staying the same. I thought I would be my daughter's anchor in that moment like my mother had been in mine.

'Fine. If you want to go then leave. We won't stand in your way if this is going to make you happy.' I said with my eyes meeting the floor we covered in carpet.

I didn't want her to see the dejection in my eyes. I would miss her laughter, our talks, heated discussions, and debates. Mostly I would miss her presence. But she was depressed. She hated school. She had done very badly in the exams. Magdalene was still alive then. So Swaziland it was then for O and A levels and then The London Film School that is if she could get a British Council scholarship if she was lucky.

My mother had been my anchor throughout my depressive episodes. The crushing highs that took me to the wuthering heights of Rhodes and London and the numbing, frustrating lows that took me to my bed. Sometimes I would just lay on the bed still in my suit.my body was not sore, did not feel tired, my eyes were burning, but sleep would not come, only a numb sensation starting from the top of me head that would make its way down to the tips of my toes. Every parent wants to protect their child, sometimes protect them from everything. The world isn't all bad. Tomorrow isn't going to be all doom and gloom like today was. There are good people in this world who are just as affected by sickness, chronic illness, cancers, diseases

Madness? Madness! What is madness? What a question! Do people question John Nash? Do they call him mad, insane, tell him that he's weird? Do they question this genius's sanity, his intelligence, or do they just write him off as wired differently from the rest of the human race. Is he an anomaly? One evening my children came to me. My son looked at me. Tall, dark, and handsome, one would be forgiven for thinking his introversion is arrogance he said, 'Dad. It's time for you to sit down and write your story. Write your memoir. Write your autobiography if you will.' To tell you the truth it has been two years now, nearly three. I can't clearly recall if that conversation ever took place. I can't remember who said what, when, the how I was going to go about it. I have written about depression. I have written about mental health. I have written books. South End. The aftermath of the forced removals. To be honest with you people didn't stand in line for me sign that book. My guess that that was a sign. A sign from God. I paid attention. I listened. And I turned my attentions elsewhere to committee meetings, reading the newspapers. People just didn't like me to talk about apartheid. That book quietly disappeared, and went out of print. People just weren't into that vibe. The book wasn't giving off good vibrations so people weren't turning up to buy that book. But out of everything that I have written so far that book is my favourite. I have written about depression before from a sufferer's perspective, and that little book turned out to be an enormous bit of loose cannon, then a diamond in the rough, and then a little gem of a book.

People like to romanticise apartheid now but I don't. They put up pictures, photographs, paintings of struggle heroes and heroines in museums. There are public holidays, streets, buildings, foundations, bursaries, books, poetry, memoirs, autobiographies named after them, written in memory of them and some of them are even given honorary doctorates. Some posthumously. All I think about these days in the autumn of my years as I watch television at night, bits and pieces of the news, well, it means absolutely nothing to me. Climate change, global warning, it's just the recession that has hit us all the hardest. My friends are no longer here. Most of them have passed on. I remember them fondly. Sometimes with tears in my eyes. I'm an old man now. I'm losing my hair. My wife, young and pretty. She will always be young and pretty to me. The blushing bride in her white lace on her wedding day. I remember I lost one of my white gloves between signing the register (I have a Scout's knot in my throat now when I think back to my wedding day. My own children won't understand this. They won't understand what married life is until my son steps over that threshold with his new wife. Until my girls have said, 'In sickness and health. Till death do us part.' Come hell or high water I will be here for them all until the day I can't be here anymore. I do what I can. I put the apron on and wash the dishes. Dry them carefully. Pack them away. The women in this house are always rearranging the furniture in the kitchen. But that has nothing to do with me. I play my part. I have a role to play in this family. I am the patriarch of this household. I am father. I am uncle. I am nurturer, caretaker, provider, and breadwinner. If we must eat pies for supper, then I walk down the road and buy them. I swing my arms. I walk much more these days than I did before but not far. Not far.) So now where was I? Right. I lost my white glove and Gerda was laughing at me. I got lucky. I didn't really deserve her you know what with everything I put her and the children through. But somehow we made it to the other side. She's angelic. She is. My wife. My wife. My wife. Abigail is the oldest and the brightest star in my universe. My Beethoven and my Kubrick. She has been through so much. Up streets and down streets. Johannesburg and Swaziland. Film school. School after school after school.

Psychometric tests. She's done them all, and they have all said the same thing. She's been psychoanalysed to death by psychologist after psychologist but she has a fighting spirit. All my children have fighting spirits. My son has done the impossible. He has given me an heir to the throne. Words can't express what I feel when I look at his son. My son. My son and his son. Abigail, well, I think she thinks too much (she's curious about everything, every impulse that the human species has, everything negative that happens in the world, the aftershocks are always of biblical proportions. I worry for her. Her personality is different. She lives by a completely different set of rules. People who live with depression often do live a life made up with a mind-set of elegant mathematics. She doesn't think like a woman. My son and daughter are both complex creatures. Their mother elegant, and cold. When she descended upon Port Elizabeth after the honeymoon she seemed so exotic, so out of place here but she soon picked out furniture for out flat. Made it comfy. We had so many plans, dreams and goals. It was very, very difficult to conceive children. It took us five years and then we had Abigail, who was followed by another short stop and then my son, my son. Ambrose, my son. He is my namesake. He is my pride and joy. All I do these days is talk, and talk, and talk. Mostly about the past before I forget. I have to remember to write down everything I say because if I forget then who will remember the forced removals, South End, Fairview (where my mother had property, a domestic worker of all people, a seamstress at one of the best high schools in the country. She saved her money for a rainy day and bought land.) I think if you want to romanticise anything don't romanticise your education, romanticise your culture, your heritage instead. Don't romanticise mental illness, your London experience, or your European experience, visits to castles, trips in gondolas, the palace of Versailles, romanticise your family life, your domestic duties. Romanticise writing. Abigail is a poet. My second daughter has done very well for herself. Well, she lives in Johannesburg, works in a bank. She's moneyed. Now she's a socialite, a connoisseur if I ever saw one. I just didn't mean to bring up one. If I don't write nobody will remember anything about the Coloured identity, psyche and intellect in the Northern Areas from my generation. We'll all be six feet under, pushing up daisies pretty soon. And then what? Ghosts. Getting a dead man to tell you a story about his childhood days is like squeezing blood from a stone. Have you ever tried squeezing blood from a stone? I remember when I was writing up my historical research about the London Missionary Society the state of mind I was in. I was on a hypomanic high while I was writing most of it. Nearing a complete collapse. I thought my professor would tell me, 'Ambrose, what is this? It's a complete and utter disaster from start to finish'. But I persevered. He's in Canada now or dead. But I give my peace wherever he is. He was a part of my life for a very long time. I appreciated all his help. He was very liberal of course in his ideas of politics of course. We would never have tea together. That's what I mean. Sometimes after driving hours from Port Elizabeth to Grahamstown. After making the trip I would make my way to his office and to my utter astonishment he would not be there. The door would be locked. It would sometimes bring tears to my eyes. Yes. He made me cry. For ten years up and down. I was principal at the time at a public school in a sub-economic area. I taught the kids there to reach for the stars. I can never seem to place names to all the faces who stop me in the street or who kindly offer me a lift home. I take their hand. And in their faces even when I don't recognise them all I see is affection, honesty, and gratitude for what I taught them, for what I said, even though I was tough on them. I sometimes took a lot of heat for what I said from Inspectors, from irate parents who would come to see after I had given their angel six of the best. There was no detention in those days. Corporal punishment wasn't abhorred as it is now. I loved those kids like I loved my three children at home. Hundreds and hundreds of them. Where are all of them now, I wonder to myself sometimes? Are they all successful? Are they making money? Are they paying their mortgages, seeing to the bills, or are they unemployed. In the good old days when we had a near perfectly run education system even in the Northern Areas (even though it was under an apartheid government run by Coloured Affairs) many of my kids made their way to universities overseas. Many of them live their now, are raising their own families there now. Many have it to easy. They're living the easy life. And they've completely erased the past. The poverty, the spiritual poverty, the hunger, the desire to learn on the faces of the children who came from much more impoverished homes. Matchstick houses we called them in those days. They're still standing in the Northern Areas to this day a symbol of racial hatred for all the world to see. Our society is traumatised. People are traumatised. The youth are affected mostly by drugs. The drug of choice these days for Coloured youth is tik. Babies having babies. More and more children being born out of wedlock. Where is this taking place? In the Northern Areas.

Chapter 3
The Difficulties of a Bride

And for every matchstick house in the burbs of the Northern Areas there's a father and a mother. There's a family in ganglands. Symbolic of apartheid. Symbolic of ethnic cleansing. Symbolic of the divide between wealth and poverty, the disenfranchised marginalised youth who have no skills. Only unemployment staring them in the face, and in the shadows. Foreshadowing every glimpse of their identity, lock, stock, and barrel. Ammunition has become like Braille is for the blind. All youth well they must be initiated into the gang. They must know how to knife, how to stab, how to make a knife, a knife that can go in for the kill. For every wedding, there's a bridal bouquet, the bride, and her wedding feast sometimes in a Methodist church hall or sometimes not. For every Baptist, Protestant, Presbyterian, Mormon, Muslim, there's an agnostic. I was lucky that I just escaped that lifestyle by the skin of my teeth while growing up in South End before we were forcibly removed by police and by the government of the day.

My son when he talks sometimes it's hard for me to follow (he has so many ideas, you see). It's hard to understand what he is talking about. He talks fast. He uses wild hand gestures a lot when he is making a point. I wish they would all come to church with me. I wish they could all be saved, baptised. But we all worship the same God. For some of us he's right here with us on this planet, beside us, walking beside us in our hour or time of need. For others like my wife God is on an astral plane. I try and understand her. Love has a delicate smell. There was a time when we had good times. We'd eat out. There'd be movie night. We'd leave the children at home and go and watch a film. But now it's different. She's a grandmother. I'm a grandfather.

Overnight we've become different people. It's as if the ordinary madness that other people call reality has possessed both of us. Times were good. Times are still good.

I remember my mother was a domestic worker. Ouma. Oupa. Both fervently borderline-religious.

I remember so many things now about my childhood with such a clarity of vision. Thought patterns come in waves. Their crests are beautiful, magnificent, electrifying, Cheshire cat magical.

Once upon a time long ago, more years than I care to remember I decided not to return to university to complete my teacher's diploma but rather to complete my B.Sc. Honours in Botany at the University of the Western Cape. I was refused admission due to my political past. I decided to teach and bank my salary in order to repay the government loan I had received in order to complete my degree. I got a teaching degree at my alma mater South End High School in January 1965. I was excited and looked forward to the challenge although my teaching roster was very loaded. For the standard sixes I had social studies and general science. I took the standard sevens for history and taught another class history in Afrikaans and then there were my standard nine classes. I taught physiology and hygiene. This was one of the main reasons which militated against me making a success of my teaching career. Many of the pupils were older than myself and I found myself teaching in the medium of Afrikaans even though I never had a teaching certificate. The students were difficult. I felt frustrated as if I could not get through to them. Of course I didn't realise I could not relate to them and they could not relate to me. For the large part they were undisciplined. Large classes made circumstances for effective teaching impossible. For the first three months I managed to cope however come to

April I started to slow down. I could not concentrate on my lesson plans and found it easier to give up. I frequently fell into fits of depression and spells of self-pity. I found it difficult to teach. I was completely disinterested and demotivated. I found myself withdrawing from social interaction at school and at home. I left for school in the morning and stayed in the classroom for the rest of the school day. There was no discipline in the classes as I said before. This made things even tougher for me. I was disorganised. The pupils carried on acting out. They did just as they pleased. Pupils ran riot all over me, I virtually dragged myself through a school day. I had no assistance or support from my colleagues or people who I considered to be my friends. I also had no appetite and could not fall asleep at night. I was like a zombie from Hollywood B-movie dragging myself to school and home and back again. The doctor diagnosed me with having a vitamin deficiency. Anxiety overwhelmed me as I fell more and more behind with my lessons. I was overtaken by guilt of the injustice I was doing my pupils. I asked myself questions like who would be responsible if the pupils had to fail their examinations. Could I blame the principal, parents, learners or myself? I now felt like I was in a bottomless pit and in a dark tunnel. This was what always wavered on my mind those days. A feeling of gloom began to overwhelm me and suicide seemed to be the only way out. My thought process slowed down almost until it came to a standstill. My mind was completely clouded with negativity. After school I would spend the majority of my time in my bedroom. I vividly remember putting a plastic bag over my head. It burst before I suffocated. My mother was the only one who stood by me during this difficult time of my life. She prayed for me and saw that I had something to eat, had clean clothing. If that was hell what was to follow was even a greater hell. The viciousness of depression lifted and symptoms in direct contrast to the previous phase prevailed. I became talkative, loud, agitated. I walk around the whole school and the vicinity where I lived. I visited and spoke to people I never knew before. Within two weeks I spent all my savings which I religiously accumulated over a period of six months on useless items like antiques, liquor, old music records. Gifts were brought for people I met for the first time and I spent no time of the person. I did not sleep at night. I had no concern for my welfare. I did not listen to the people who had my best interests at heart. I could not bring myself to eat anything and walked long distances. Up streets and down streets. I decided to walk along the National Road to Cape Town. The road was pitch dark. This did not matter since I had a lot of energy. I got a lift in a furniture truck as far as Swellendam and then proceeded to the Meyer family in Bellville South. Two ministers of the United Congregational Church had me admitted as a voluntary patient at the Valkenburg Psychiatric Hospital in Pinelands Cape Town. For the first time I realised that I was in a mental institution when on admission I was given a polo jersey, khaki shorts and a pair of sandals. I was placed in a locked up ward. The patients came from all walks of life and suffered from all forms of mental illness. I was not diagnosed with any mental illness however I was not released from the locked up ward. However I must admit that it was therapeutic to be among other mentally ill sufferers. However I missed Port Elizabeth and my family. After a month at Valkenburg Psychiatric Hospital I took my leave to the medical school at Groote Schuur where I wanted to be in the first place. I then meandered through District Six where I found families dismantling their homes and belongings as a result of the forced removals of 1965.These residents were being moved to the Cape Flats and areas like Mitchell's Plan, Lavenderhill. These are now the centres of gang warfare. I sought help from the social worker at Groote Schuur Hospital. They supplied me with cigarettes, pocket money, and a third class railways ticket to Port Elizabeth. On the train I discovered that I had left the ticket in the jacket I had loaned while in Cape Town. Therefore I had no ticket on the train with the result that the guard and the policeman wanted to put me off the train at the next station. They were reluctant to believe my explanation. When reaching Port Elizabeth they handed me over to the police where I had to sign an undertaking that I would pay the cost of the ticket as I began teaching again.

Then I had a manic episode in Kimberly. My services had terminated at the South End High School. In January 1966 I was offered a temporary post at a high school in Square Hill Park in Kimberly. I made a grave mistake by not checking on my medication. There was no psychiatrist or doctor who could describe mood stabilising drugs. I arrived in Kimberly on the 1st of February. The first month went okay. I gave my lessons clearly and meaningfully then all hell broke loose. I experienced a major episode of mania. I could not stop myself from making grave errors in judgement. I took myself to teach on a Saturday morning. During which time I consumed excessive amounts of whisky and milk. I spend long hours at school disturbing other teachers in the classrooms. I was creating complete mayhem in the school. I was not prepared to listen to the advice of well-meaning individuals. I also took to drinking alcohol. My meagre salary militating it becoming an uncomfortable habit. I spent a daily visit to the Kemo Hotel. I shudder to reflect on my manic state during the inter-Provincial swimming tournament of the Swimming Federation of South Africa. All the provinces from all over South Africa took part. I took charge of all the arrangements of the tournament, although I had no knowledge of competitive swimming. It was a disaster from the start. Without anybody's permission I appointed myself the manager of the Griqua Team. This was extremely embarrassing to the rest of the Griqua officials. I placed myself in charge of the bus which was going to transport teams and officials to a holiday resort along the Vaal River. I waded into the children's swimming pool in my pants and vest vainly trying much to the amusement of the crowd. I visited a family in Kimberly and was attracted by their son's toy gun which resembled a real gun. I went around the area and scared people as if it was a real gun. People began to avoid me as the stigma of mental illness was pronounced.

There's nothing sexy about having a recurring mental illness like it's portrayed in American films. Some people you can trace its origins along your family tree. Some say it's in the nucleic acid of the ladders of your genes, your biochemistry. Maybe your dendrites are just out of sync with the dopamine and serotonin levels in your brain for that cycle, or season, or day. Maybe you were just having a stressful day. Mental illness is governed by equal measures of loss, feeling shattered, truth feels sharp, you become aware of the isolation you might feel from time to time, acutely aware of the environments and the landscape you find yourself in, and intense mourning that can startle you out of your reverie. Mind you, it is not who you. And it does not define who you are as a person, your character, or your personality. It doesn't matter what 'they' say. They don't have your psychiatrist's degree behind their name. You're human. Pain is what comes along with the territory of humanity. Understand it, learn from it, navigate those 'shark-infested' (or should I say stigma-busting) dangerous waters with your moral compass. This earth is damaged. We are damaged. Damaged people. Shattered. As I've said before we live in a traumatised country. The entire fabric of society is traumatised. The nuclear family as a unit is traumatised. So now we have to learn how to survive. How do the mentally ill, the most displaced, the most embarrassed, largely the most ridiculed, and humiliated respond to survival? Instinct. From my perspective we all have to rely on it at some point in our lives. And it works every time. Just remember you have to swim before you begin to tread upon land. And if at first you don't succeed, try and try and try again. You can mourn the fact that now that you are aging, this also means becoming more comfortable with your principles, more in tune with virtuous qualities as you grow older, you are also becoming wiser, more understanding of your mental illness, your relapses, your recovery. Yes, some people who are mentally ill hear voices. That is as scary for them as it is for you. Some people see things, have hallucinations, and it is very real for them. That is as scary for them as it is for you. Some men, though mostly women who are mentally ill can became promiscuous seeing it as a replacement for real intimacy and unconditional love that they should have received from their parents in the first place. Know that you belong in this word whether you have a disability, mental illness, or have refugee status. Know that having a mental illness doesn't mean self-punishment, or self-imposed exile. You have one life to live. It is precious. So why not start now. Don't let your mental illness feed you, scar you, wound you intrinsically speaking, sate you, starve you. If you are mentally ill you have the right not to hurt yourself, but you do have the right to accept yourself, love all of who you are unconditionally. People might think you're not good enough, thin enough, pretty enough, but that is just an opinion. Determining if the glass is half full (positive vibrations switch on), or of its half empty (negative vibes switch off). Your conscious mind speaks to your subconsciousness mind all the time.

In April 1966 I returned to Port Elizabeth. My mania had abated and I obtained a temporary teaching post at the Gelvandale Secondary School. It was located in Helenvale which was a sub economic area and was established as a result of the slum clearance scheme of the municipality and the government. The area was soon overcrowded three primary and one secondary school was built in the space of three years. Ten people had to use one outside toilet. The streets were scattered with litter and dirt. The pupils came mainly barefoot to school and without any lunch. My class had more than 60 children. There were insufficient desks and writing materials. These circumstances made my teaching days in the beginning difficult, sad and depressing.

I had taken Zoology as one of my degree subjects. I collected stray cats. I placed one on a glass sheet which I covered with a bell jar and placed chloroform on wadding and placed it under the bell jar. I had underestimated the strength of the drugged cat.

In November 1966, the year mark for General Science and Social Studies had to be prepared for moderation by the Inspector of Education. At that time I fell into another deep episode. I slowed down, demotivated to do the simplest of tasks. I felt deep exhaustive depression. In the absence of the principal the deputy showed no sympathy for my depression. The day before the Inspector arrived my work was not yet complete yet the Inspector Mr Swanepoel ordered me to leave the school immediately despite the explanation of my depression. Fortunately for me the principal had just arrived from Cape Town. He assessed the situation, told me to see a doctor and to return to teaching when I felt well again. As I left the school to board the bus I was overwhelmed by suicidal thoughts. I had a strong desire for the bus to crash. This was not to be. I was alone at home and decided to take an overdose of tablets. It turned out to have the opposite effect. It didn't even make me drowsy or sleepy. The tablets that I did take turned out to be too few to have a serious effect. I got to the Port Elizabeth Mental Health Society where I received help.

Suicide was uppermost in my mind to the extent that I was continually thinking about taking an overdose of tablets. Fortunately my mother's early return from work removed these negative thoughts from my mind.

I was taken to the humble offices of the Port Elizabeth Mental Health Society in Brassell Street in North End where the social workers in particular Jann Hollingshead spent almost three hours of therapy with me so I could realise that suicide was not the only way out in a crisis situation. The next day I had an appointment with the psychiatrist in the outpatient department of the Livingstone hospital. He diagnosed me with manic depression also known as bipolar mood disorder. The seriousness of my condition necessitated five sessions of electroconvulsive therapy. A white patch had to be applied to both sides of my head which got me the nickname of the Western actor Jack Palance. I felt very sore and hurt when I heard these remarks made by people who I thought were my friends. I was also very young. I had never heard of electroconvulsive therapy before. Since I was not aware of what it was I was very apprehensive at every occasion when I had to receive the treatment. However the white doctor who was in his fifties explained to me that the seriousness of my major depressive episode necessitated this treatment. He also gave me the assurance that the treatment wasn't a guarantee that I was to recover. I didn't know what the hell was going on the day I left the hospital that day. I was twenty years old. I don't know when I fell in love with Jann. She was vivacious. But I knew that nothing would ever come of it. She died of throat cancer. August died of stomach cancer. Jean died of breast cancer. Cancer riddled bodies. Cancer riddled cells. I imagined the white bloods cells putting up a fight, while the cancer cells still got through floating by them like free radicals to attack the golden cells of organs and tissue. People die every day. Every Saturday churches are packed. Parking lots filled with cars.

People coming to pay their respects. And sometimes I was one of them. Shaking people's hands firmly. Looking them in the eye and saying, 'My condolences to you and your family. I am really sorry for your loss.' And I really meant it. I really did. Present day. Keep up or you'll get lost. Jann's loss. I never quite got over that. She was still so young. She could have had that sunny road. I could have met her on that sunny road. Perhaps we could have had those kids, a family, raised them in England. Perhaps she asked for me when she was in the hospital. If I had gone it would have meant a sense of closure on both of parts. I don't think I have ever loved a woman, known a woman like Jann Hollingshead so intimately just from our conversations. Love has a delicate smell. Hospitals smelled of furniture polish, nail polish remover, something antiseptic, and sanitary. I know standing next to her bed watching while she slept, or drift in and out of consciousness, I would have perhaps lost all sense of self-control, my belief in God, or perhaps we both would have found closure. But I wanted to remember her smile, handing over the 'contraband', my favourite brand of cigarettes (how did she remember), and us tucking into the purest pub lunch you could find in England, and meeting Jann's sister and computer programmer husband in their lovely home. The feeling of being invited, this grand gesture, how excited I was to explore the city of London. I felt like Sir Arthur Conan Doyle's Sherlock Holmes. From the beginning of childhood I always felt cast out of society. But in London town I was a new man (Jann's man? No. I had decided. I had made up my mind that Gerda was the only woman for me. And if it wasn't for her, for Abigail, for short stop, for Ambrose, for Cody, for Ethan, for Lauren, I wouldn't be the man that I am today if it wasn't for my angels). But sometimes I think to myself of Columbia University. I would have been a unique 'Christopher Columbus'-type don't you think striding not sprinting? Sometimes I think of that sunny road. Sometimes I think a lot of Jann. How I let her go without even saying goodbye. That wasn't very gentlemanly of me because I had thought very highly off her, and she of me.

In 1974 I won a scholarship by the British Council to complete a study of the mentally and physically handicapped in England and Wales and implement it in the position in South Africa. It was a very valuable scholarship since it covered a return plane ticket, tuition fees, books, warm clothing and even a maintenance grant. I was very happy, excited and content to undertake the scholarship and complete the relevant study. All went well up to the Christmas recess when the English students went home for the holidays. I with my friend, Jones Mceke and other African students was left behind to make provision for ourselves. I took the opportunity to organise a trip via Cosmos travel agency to visit five or six of the European countries. This was a dream come true for me since I visited Brussels in Belgium, Cologne and Frankfurt in Germany, Florence, the Vatican, Rome, Paris and then back via Dover. One of the most remarkable incidents happened to me at the customs at Dover. I was placed in a room with my luggage where I was asked to open my cases so that the customs officials could search my clothing. They also asked me a number of questions concerning my place of origin, why I had come to London and when I was going to return to South Africa again. After about two hours I was allowed to go. I then bordered the train to Euston Station which was not far from the residence. I was very, very down, depressed and sad at the happening at Dover. And I just wanted to go home to South Africa, however my friend Jones was waiting for me. He helped me with my luggage and got me to my room. I realised that a major episode of depression was on its way. I had no appetite. I was exhaustibly tired. I couldn't fall asleep and I didn't know what to do because just before I left a young black student from Kenya who was manic depressive was sent home without getting suitable treatment. I thought that the same fate would face me. I couldn't get up out of bed in the morning. And I only responded to persistent knocking of my friend Jones. He got me out of bed. He saw to it that I got dressed and washed and virtually forced me to go to a nearby restaurant where I could enjoy some breakfast. I felt much better after that but not good enough. He took me back to my room where he sorted my clothing and placed the dirty clothing in a bag and took me to a Laundromat where he saw to it that I washed my clothing. Jones saved me. I wouldn't be sitting where I am today, surrounded by a loving and supportive family and my first grandchild, my son's son if it wasn't for Jones Mceke. Jones not only saw to my physical needs but was always encouraging and motivating me to allow the dark clouds of negativity and depression to lift. Fortunately when the university reopened I felt much better and could take my meals in the canteen and attend lectures as well as school visit in the English countryside. I must emphasise that I really enjoyed the greenery of the countryside. I will never forget my trip from London to Glasgow on the Express that travelled from the one end of England to the rest of Glasgow in Scotland. For the first time I could appreciate where English literary figures and poets could get their inspiration. London. Walking up streets, and down streets. The young man who had the dorm room next to mine always invited his friends over for coffee but I was never invited. He was a minister, what they call a pastor now. He never talked to me. Never once looked in my direction. But there were people who were kind. Kinder to me I think because they see I was depressed. Michelle, Sue, Jan, my memories of madness, my education at the school of life, religion, Bush University, and eventually I found that perpetual balance I had been searching for my whole life. I found that balance in my community work, my bright faith, the respect, loyalty and love I had for my wife, the affection I had for my children. The memories of my family coming to visit me at

Hunterscraig Psychiatric Clinic are bright in my mind. My children were still very small. My wife and I would whisper to each other while they played, so innocent on the far side of the garden. They would hug and kiss me before they left. It broke my heart to see their heads at the back of the car waving madly goodbye to me. My son, my son, his hair dark and curly, already his mother's favourite. The girls would cling to each other waiting for me to get up grass stains on my pants, helping my wife get up who put her best smile, her best foot forward. My oldest, oh-so-serious in the seat in front with her mother and the middle child with a Cheshire cat smile saying, 'We'll see you soon daddy. See you tomorrow.' Every year or so this was repeated. Hospitalisation followed by recovery, then a relapse, and very soon my children grew up and they weren't affectionate children anymore. Instead they became rebellious, anxious teenagers who often could not find the words to describe what they were feeling and thinking. I missed the days of their innocence like I missed my years at the Bush University.

When it comes to mania I'm a wreck. When it comes to depression I go kaput. I can only see the tunnel of light cutting through the periphery of my vision. The tunnel of light you see when you have a near death experience. Sometimes depression can be like that. Fluid multiplying. Make you think about things that happened to you as a child. Traumatic things that you'd rather not to be thinking about. You'd rather find yourself making love, you know. Or eating barbecue at the beach.

Chapter 4
The Ambitious Man

And then you find yourself inside of a dream. Quite literally, and figuratively a dream world.

We never did get around to building the swimming pool in our backyard that my wife and I often spoke about. We said it would be for the children, for the children. Instead the swimming pool could never be built because there were pipes underneath running under the ground where we wanted it to go. So ideas for swimming lessons were planted inside my wife's head. Mine too. Romance! What a harsh experience. Love, the interlude between two acts. Oh how it changes everything about the world experience, materialism, values, spiritual poverty, and that prime commodity of all commodities, spirituality. When I became a writer, I didn't really know how I was going to go about it. Didn't know really what I was getting myself into. But my wife stood by me. Saw me through that manic phase as well. I need her. I still need her by my side. Her elegance, her humour, and her beauty is what gets me through the day. I need her like grit. The strange thing is she will always be good enough for me, but will I be good enough for her? What can get this bleak pose out of me, this dogged depression, this fierce, fatal memory? I will remember my wife always as the exotic Gerda that I brought home to my mother, my father, sisters, and my brothers. How I will remember that this romance will live long, and will go on, and on, and on. She will remain beautiful to me now and forever more, even in old age.

Careful not to spill your warm soda, handling plates carefully on your knees, surrounded by your family, faces of love, your children, your wife. So this is my story. This is it. This is where it all began seventy years ago. I am an old man now. I am a man who is in the autumn of his years. I'm a father who is looking at his son's proud, and handsome face. He is embracing his namesake, my grandchild, my grandson, our legacy. Standing by his side is the beautiful, high-spirited young woman he has decided to take as his life-partner. He has the wisdom I did not have at his age. All I feel now is infirmity humming in my bones like never before. A chronic fatigue that descends upon me in the mornings like never before. The years that I was a young, virile man are gone. Have I left too much to fate in my own children's lives? Should I have protected them more when I had the chance? I am left to wonder. They have all surpassed the dreams I have had for them. Abigail has surrendered everything to the universe. She is a poet and a writer. Ambronese has made a success of her life. In everything she has set out to do. She works in a bank as a research strategist. Ambrose is a businessman involved in playing at local politics the same position I found myself decades ago as a young man at the Bush University. Well, all three of them didn't have the longing I did to have a London experience. Ambronese, has travelled a great deal. India, Thailand, North America. My pilgrimage came with running with scissors, impressions on student life at Western Cape, surveying the landscape that was London, winter trees in London, the long road to spirituality, and so I made gods out of my education at Bush University, UNISA, Rhodes, and London University. I worshiped the buildings behind those tall gates, and cathedral-like inspired spires. I found myself in London. Escaping from the wuthering heights of apartheid South Africa. Steve Biko's Azania. I would look at White people in their perfumed European world, their airs and graces, the fat of the land on their lips. Fruit, olive oil, pasta, and tomatoes in their trolleys in the shiny aisles their supermarkets. Of course it wasn't home to me. This new strange land. And standing next to me was my friend, Mr. Jones. He became, in that year, my brother and anchor that cemented me, planted me in this foreign land's soil, and what still resides to this day in my heart besides our friendship, were the walls of those gardens made of stone, and everything that was healing. It was stick fighting days for me all over again. The hell of childhood trauma (the bullying on the playground, those playing fields). Selling peanuts. Selling newspapers for peanuts. A forest of pain tearing into me, through me on fire as I felt my father's belt. Black is not ugly. It is something quite quietly, and remarkably beautiful inside and out. It's a river running through all of us. Through this life force of a nation. Hemingway had Europe. Ambrose Cato George had London, had half of the world at his feet, and beside him he had Mceke Jones, the best friend, the best man that anybody could ask for. A comrade. He had a face as dark as an orchard at night, as night land, a postcard of war, the blurred lines on the gravestones in a cemetery through tears of suffering or rain, an oceans' tides and currents rising up to meet a physical body of sea mist. And every dress that I saw in a shop's window in London I pictured Gerda in it, when we'd be reconciled. Together again in each other's company I convinced myself that would give me renewed strength, and vigour, and the depression would no longer dog me, terrify me. Mceke Jones pictured my suffering although I can imagine that in his own way he did not have the words for it. But something inside of him made him feel empathy for the condition he sometimes found me in in the mornings. When I was beside myself, could not make it to breakfast in the canteen, it was Mr. Jones who saw to it that I had something to eat. He was a lovely man. I have never met anyone quite like him again in my life. He must have had a wonderful mother. Well, we never spoke much about our childhood dreams. I had just seen the advertisement in the newspaper by chance for scholarships to study abroad. I don't even think we got around to asking each other how on earth we met under the circumstances we did.

It's lovely to dream. I would literally be in bed under the covers, and think hours away much to the consternation of the Portuguese cleaning lady who made the rooms in the dormitory tidy. I was in her way. She was in my personal space. I didn't want to return to Gerda like that. A broken man. Wherever Mceke Jones is, I think he must be safely tucked away in a high position in government, or in retirement surrounded by his children and grandchildren, adored, highly inspiring his sons and daughters, his grandchildren to follow in his footsteps, to have that London experience. And I wonder to myself did he have that sunny road? Did he have rain on his wedding day? Did he swim in the sea with his wife, ever take his wife to the moveable feast of Paris, Hemingway's Paris? Still I wonder about all of my dreams, all of the goals I've had. I've achieved much. Plenty. I've achieved my potential, and then some. And other men, and women? Are they happy? Are they fulfilled when they look around themselves? Are they sated? Or are they sad, do they feel frustrated, downcast, or do they cast aspersions on other people? People well I see them every day. They walk past me with smiles on their faces or a downcast look in their eyes and I tell myself secretly that there's a story there. There's a love story, or that person is haunted by something (perhaps by some of the same things that I was haunted by). And I look at my daughters, a young poet, and a young woman who works in a bank. I produced that. They're walking around with my genes in them. Their offspring will have (there's a good chance that it will happen) my genes in them. This makes me happy, but it also makes me sad. And here is where my story begins to unfold. I saved the best of me till last. For my grandson Ethan. The heir to the throne. For my children, my beautiful wife, my daughter-in-law. This, this book is for you. Always remember that there is loveliness in the world around you, that the genius's behaviour can exist for long periods in loneliness, and solitude, their vulnerability sometimes aches for company, that there is an internal struggle in both the introvert and the extrovert. Both can become the hypomanic leader, entrepreneur, and even the educationalist (as I once was), and particularly the actor. And so I come to my swan song. We live in a traumatic society. The fabric of the universe is changing as fast as the advances we are making in technology. Someday perhaps that technology will surpass humanity (although I pray that it doesn't). Geniuses are always on a journey. People journey all the time. Some find themselves in self-imposed exile. Some travel to India, far off places where they can find themselves, journey within, discover themselves through meditation, self-discovery, self-actualisation, through that phenomena, that reality, and that nature. But the fact of the matter is we are all born geniuses. What we do with that gift, that potential isn't always up to us though as I discovered in my own life. I hope you will come to realise that like the genius you are always on a journey from spiritual poverty to a journey of self-discovery.

This is my story. A memory of madness. Of suffering in silence. One man's fable is another man's parable is another man's perspective in the flesh across a wilderness history carrying a survival guide with him. He hasn't got his whole future ahead of him mapped out just yet. He can't believe yet that he's just met the woman he's going to spend the rest of his life with. That they will be excited on their wedding day, but that their marriage will have its highs, and lows. This diary of madness is in praise of my mother. Her wisdom. There's an insanity that borders on modern day humanity's unquiet mind. An insanity that is never spoken of. When I grew up, some might say how that it was an idyllic childhood, but there was also an insanity that bordered on the Cheshire cat in Alice in wonderland. And so what was happening on the rest of the African continent became either a dream or a nightmare. But it made no sense to me. It never reached my understanding, my sensibility, and the fragments of human bodies in war, reconciliation, and peace in the African Renaissance, the duplicity of the promulgation of the Group Areas Act, and Post Traumatic Stress Disorder. The revolution (if ever there was one taking place at the height of White South Africa, at those wuthering heights of apartheid South Africa, was a revolution that was more of an unseen movement at the least. A revolution from within (like its counterpart in the West, feminism). Although women at the time of apartheid weren't as liberated as their counterparts in the West. In life there are always choices. Sometimes you make the right life choices, and this brings you pleasure, but sometimes they bring you pain. And sometimes from lonely, humiliating experiences there will come a dream that you will never completely wake up from. Like marriage, a good woman who doesn't believe in wearing sensible shoes. Goals can become as stale as a loaf of bread, that stuck record, leaving one eternally morally bankrupt, and sounds which were once familiar to each other like a man and woman embracing each other in front of their children, their muffled 'I love you,' hidden from view, and you will begin to realise that love it changing everything once again in its path. Always hidden from view it is working from the outside, its private domain. There's creativity in everything around you, particularly in sufferers of mental illness. At the end of the day whether you have a mental illness, experience a profound measure of loss, of longing to belong, we are all volcano dreamers. We have a bright faith that we transfer onto our children. I knew when and where I was not welcome, although it was difficult for me to realise it at the time in my most lucid moments. There was always the ballad of life to keep me company into the early hours of the morning, and so I became a man who became the curator of his children's dreams. I think of my childhood friends. I think of them often. I miss them. You don't get to travel light in this world if you have a mental illness. Flight from the illumined glare pharmaceuticals. Flight from the illumination of pain. Flight, flight, flight, is all that you can think of when illness descends.

I saw the early death of a man in my father's eyes every day as I grew up from a young boy into a man. I saw the early death of men in my childhood friends. One by one they have crossed over to the hereafter, eternity. Soon I will be with them too. I have to make peace with that. I have lived. I had that love story after all. Searching for longing on a shoestring budget is something you will never forget. I will never forget Arthur Nortje, Dennis Brutus, Frank Landman, and my years as a student, and then as a teacher at my alma mater South End High School in Walmer (a suburb filled with townhouses and developers wanting to build more town houses). Women have always inspired me. My mother, my wife, some of the women I have taught with, even my own daughters. I have grown to respect their own ideas, sometimes foolhardy, and as a father I have always forgiven them of the mistakes that they have made. All the women who have inspired, Jann for instance, have been both fiercely loyal to me and fiercely intelligent. I remember my own teachers with a great amount of fondness. How distant those dizzy plans of London seem now? I have lived with manic depression for fifty years now. I've come this far. How far do I still need to go? I look at Gerda. Night land has descended upon her garden. She is waiting for the moon to come out stars like birds in her eyes. Her throat hidden by a scarf to keep her warm. My daughter, my eldest with her bohemian customs, writing rituals, talks to me of a Salvation Army mattress, the brief flame of fame, and how it crushed her. Is crushing her? She doesn't yet that all of that is her imagination's brief respite. She doesn't yet know that in order to make art, you have to live it too. And in the early hours of the morning when I get up, and make my way to the kitchen I don't think of my children as damaged and dysfunctional (although throughout their adolescence they must have felt that way sometimes). I don't know when it all came undone for all of us as a family. The moon's disappeared again. I now have joined my wife outside, alongside our eldest daughter. We have to write down affirmations about what we would like to happen in our lives and bury it in the garden. If I am going to survive a good while longer for Ethan, my grandson. If I am to cherish what I have now, it's not just hope that I must have on my side, but other things too. Of course there are things like ghosts. But they have passed on too. I have to study the survival of other writers. I fell in love with Hemingway as a young adolescent. Something in his writing freed something inside of me at first tentatively, then it became something of a catalyst. What sparked the blues death in me was all those doctors educated guesswork behind suicidal depression, and suicidal illness.

Rain is pure, and liquid. It is a ghostlike fluid blurring all the pointy edges of my sharp, shark-infested world. Walking around the house in the dead of night, switching on lights, on and off, on and off, like that mental switch in my brain, it comes back. My childhood, with such clarity, the first visit to PEMHS, and the first social worker I ever spoke to about my illness, my physical wellbeing, and the first time I tried to commit suicide by taking my father's epileptic medication. It comes back. It always comes back to me. It will always be the death of me. And I imagined that sometimes, just sometimes I must smell like death, like ill health in the early hours of the morning. At night sometimes when the children were asleep we would close our bedroom door, and remember the times when there weren't anxious, rebellious young adults in our house. Gerda would wrap her legs in blankets and I would open a bottle of sparkling wine. We would toast each other, laughing like children, behaving like a proper girlfriend, and boyfriend, happy to be alive, in each other's company, grateful for everything that had brought us together in the beginning of our relationship. We would pour the warm champagne (not real champagne of course, on a teacher's salary that would be too expensive) into glasses careful not to disturb the rest of the house. And so we communicated the anticipatory desire for each other. We were still young then. Everything in my world would be a paradise. Now although we have moves worlds apart from each other. The love is still there. That bond has grown stronger. She's planted flags though. I've planted some too. She's won prizes for it. So have I figuratively speaking. I always knew at the end of the day I will still have someone to come home too. She would still have her soul, her spirit, her kindness, and so would I although the paths that we now travelled were so different. She was searching for self-discovery through having a religious experience. I had my own quest through spirituality. Bells will be ringing. Cicadas singing but I know somehow that I won't be here forever. Out of the blue-black I will return to the black. But for now I eat my daughter's tuna fish sandwiches that she's prepared. I read her beautifully sad stories. How she weaves, and threads them. I watched Gerda braid the girls' hair when they were little. How she taught my daughters to dwell in the sunshine of possibility. How she raised a man. She did it effortlessly. She did it well. She did it to the best of her possibility. I never called my wife, 'Honey.' Too American. Besides I am not an American. I was always finding myself in a thicket in dreams, a desert filled with shrub, a forest at night, tigers burning bright. What was my subconscious trying to tell me, warn me against? I had wisdom. People would always be telling me that. When I was younger all I saw was regret. Quaint images of regret (although I never harboured any bitterness towards anyone, and I am glad that foundation was never set in stone). I needed the bright, brave, and beautiful Gerda at my side.

She made me suave, and charismatic. But that is a man far away in the mists of time. A man with golden notebooks filled with scrawl, diaries, therapy, Sundays, last nights, this morning (one of the better ones), a man standing in the rain burning with an unknown desire in his heart.

I never saw my wife as a possession. I saw her as a dream. And every day I would live inside a dream. It engulfed me like a wave. And I am glad that I that although I did take her for granted, that I never saw her as a possession. 'Look at me.' She seems to be saying all the time. 'Acknowledge me. Haven't I given you the best years of my life (take my word for it that I did, because is their other way that I can show you), my youth, three children, and now a grandchild, a daughter-in-law, and even though I was insecure sometimes I did try. I tried to love you in the best possible way I could. The best way I knew how. I loved you Ambrose Cato George unconditionally, with all my heart. Your funny, warm, sweet, and wise personality. What saved you in the end was not the therapist's chair darling. It was me. Me. Standing at your side. Driving you to your doctor's appointment. Waiting for you patiently in the car reading gardening magazine. Looking at those flowers, those tress, and imagining myself planting other versions of them in my garden. Bored out of mind, but knowing that I had to do this for you. This is what a wife does. She makes sacrifices while you live. While you're doing a mad dance, she lives quietly in her world. A wife does these things splendidly, with determination, with an art. She watches over you. She hovers. And when she is tired, she must be forgiven when she does this. Always remember to forgive me because the days when she can't do it anymore, when I couldn't do anymore for you, she doesn't simply ask her daughters, and her son to step in, your wife, me, me, me, went kaput. I could not go on forever just sacrificing all the time, giving in to your every hypomanic whim and fancy, I will and I did hand over the reins of your madness to your insecure children. It was time that they grew up. Whether I decided this, or your children did it for me, well, perhaps we'll never know. We'll never be the wiser for it. But know this. I will love you, always and forever. You are the best thing that I did, that ever happened to me. I love you Ambrose Cato George with your Ph.D., and all. I took it. I stood by you. Never forget that. So what if I peeled that hypomanic din off your planet, off your world at large. You grinned chief and beared it when I couldn't. Thank God for that. For the role that religion played in our lives. I couldn't wait to hurt, to hurt you so badly sometimes that it would turn you into a wreck, and make every nostalgic feeling that was ever there between us, I just wanted to erase it all, watch it evaporate into thin air, diminish, diminish, diminish. Forgive me. You were my silver lining more than once. I am truly sorry that I could not do more. Was I not strong enough? I don't know. This is a wife making reparations. I come to you asking you to wash away my sins. I ask your forgiveness for all the meanness I've put on display like furniture, or mannequins that left you feeling pins and needles. I took you on as a diamond in the rough. And I guess the price that both of us paid for that was very high. But I remember when I met you. I remember how we fell in love. That feeling, suddenly I was reminded that I was alive. And I realised that you can recover from grief, but you can die of heartache. And those hypomanic highs that you described to me, I could never understand them. All the reading material you gave to me highlighting depression, highlighting mania, I tried to understand how you could feel high, and depressed at the same time. I really tried. Making valiant effort after valiant effort. How could you not see how much you meant to me really in the end of every relapse, every recovery? I was always there with the children waiting to pick up the pieces, the beautiful material of our life together, and our family life together. I never left your side for a minute. But I am growing old too now. Time catches up with all of us, especially women, and sometimes it is not kind. But when I see you with the baby in your arms, our grandson, and the way you never were, or were with your children, I feel a glow, all the dreams I had for myself, my goals I had for the children, and I think about how I couldn't take the third wheel in this relationship anymore. How I couldn't take you on, your despair, your constant what seemed like commitment to me then desolation, was I a good wife to you Ambrose? I wanted it all to be perfect. Not the way my parents were together. I wanted to be happy. I wanted to feel fulfilled. Love like a sonnet your diary of madness became mine. I took it head under feet. Please try and understand this. That through it all I loved you madly. I loved you like a poet, mother, daughter, or is it hard for you to make sense out of all that I am saying. I worship you, still do although it may be hard for you to see, or read on the surface of things whenever there is tension there, that the love is still there. On the lines of your face, your wrinkled brow, the age spots, your thinning hair, and sometimes I remember the mad dance of our love, and the good times. We overcame the impossible challenges set before us. We lived through it, we loved, and laughed through it all. Smiles on our faces. We raised three beautiful, and confident human beings, who sometimes feel insecure, have the same doubts we had when we grew up. This, perhaps this is a love letter to you. In a mirror I see a wife, and babies. A Johannesburg girl has become a woman in another time, and place. Made the customary adjustments to her novel environment, her personality, the culture that she now finds herself in. I am that girl, a newlywed, and I am cleaning my house. For now, it's a flat, but I've become a woman who wants beautiful things. Expensive things. I will become a woman who saves enough money to buy the land on which her husband will build a large enough house to raise a family in. Birthdays, Christmases, Easters with pickled fish and hot cross buns will be celebrated there. And in those beginning years we will be blissfully happy, never knowing when the juggernaut of manic depression will hit. Life will become too much reduced to stream of consciousness like writing, big steps, gigantic leaps of faith, our spirituality will grow from strength to strength. And for the most of our married life we will live inside of a dream. We have to in order to survive. I love you. Do you believe it? Say you believe it. Look at me. Age has not diminished the love that I feel for you, and it never will. Your flesh and your spirit are one with nature. As we all are the bride of nature, as is humanity, I am yours Ambrose, forever.' These are words that perhaps Gerda thinks. She still acknowledges her love for me in countless ways that she can never imagine. But I do. I do. So I sit composed in the garden for what seems like hours but is only really twenty minutes with the dogs at my feet. What do I feel? What am I thinking about? Am I really happy, fulfilled, blissfully recalcitrant, satisfied, with what life offered me? Yes, yes, yes, yes, a thousand times. I have no regrets. I do not have a bitter heart. I have always believed in my children. They have taken on the world, as I took on the dangerous, oftentimes brutal, less forgiving world (what I mean to say by that is more forgiving parents). My children have taken on the world magically. Wonderfully. They've transformed it, and not the other way around. Love pours out of me for all of them. For my family, that life world, and humanity. See it seems to say to me that after all the misgivings I've had I've done the impossible. Humanity seems to say to me as I stare at my reflection in the mirror, 'Haven't turned out all that tragic after all. You've just been a comedy of errors one after the other. You've turned out like an elegantly well done sum.'

Chapter 5
Childhood

I was bom on 9 November 1944 in South End, Port Elizabeth. I was the second youngest of three brothers and two sisters. My father was a member of the Cape Corps regiment. He fought for queen and country in the Second World War. As a result of pressure in the army, he returned home after the war in a condition of ill health. The rest of his working days he spent working as a barman. Because of the long hours of his occupation, he was seldom at home. Further resentment was caused when, after his return from the Second World War, he received promises of a home and other fringe benefits from the then Jan Smuts Government. In the end all he had received was an army coat and a bicycle. Whites received homes, jobs and other fringe benefits.

My mother came from a farm called Kruisfontein, in the district of Humansdorp. She had very little formal education and was forced to work as a domestic servant for white families. She had the onerous task of bringing up 5 children. She had to play the role of mother and father because my father was for all intents the purposes and absent father. Although we were a poor family, we were held together by a very strong religious bond.

I had to carry out my responsibilities as any member of the family. My task was to buy the groceries, meat and vegetables at the cheapest possible prices in South End. This was the times an arduous but challenging task. I had to peep in at the many shops through the streets of South End, always on the lookout for a bargain. I vividly remember walking barefoot with short pants with tattered green bag under my arm buying bruised tomatoes at Damoo and fish and chips at CR Pillay. We grew up humbly and simply but were healthy and clean.

There were no extra finances to provide pocket money. I scavenged the lanes and open spaces of South End to collect old bones and bottles to earn an extra penny. These were sold for the odd tickey and sixpence at the hardware store called Finro. When I became older, I became a newspaper vendor. I sold the weekend newspaper, the Evening Post, on a fix route in the more affluent part of South End. A full recreational program augmented this. We played cricket, rugby, and soccer in the street and in the more suitable open spaces in South End.

I entered high school at the South End High School at the tender age of 12 years. It was a traumatic experience since most of my fellow pupils were older and bigger than I. This made me very timid and fearful of my peers. I continued with my menial chores and newspaper vending but I became more aware of the haves and the have-nots. Why had I to sell newspapers in the wind or rain to customers in their bright and shiny cars?

I must point out that we were a harmonious, cosmopolitan community in South End. There was little or no racial and cultural friction.

I went to school when I was only years old, which had a concomitant result that I was not psychologically ready for school and suffered as a result at all the key stages of my schooling and later university career. Through the sacrifices of my parents and older brothers and sisters, I rose above my circumstances and received a religious and ample school education. I matriculated at the age of 16 years and was forced to attend the University College of the Western Cape. The Nationalist Government had deemed it necessary that each population group had to receive their university education at their own university.

Although I wanted to become a medical doctor, and was accepted as a medical student at the University of Cape Town, I was forced due to financial restraints to forgo that and follow a teacher's course at the University of the Western Cape, since the state gave financial assistance for the course.

School and the George Family
Growing up in South End, what was intimidating was when I went to school when I was 41/2. Throughout those years it had a psychological disadvantage, particularly when I was a teenager. At age 12 I entered high school and matriculated at age 16, and went to university at age 17.
I attended a mixed race mission school, where children of all the cultural groups attended the teacher in the day school would be your Sunday school teacher. Christian hymns and prayers were said at assembly without any objection of the parents.

The church was also used as a classroom. Lunch time, bread with peanut butter and jam with milk and seasonal fruit was served during the winter months it was soup. We would line with our mugs and there was must jostling fun and laughter as we waited our turn at lunch time. During break the street was cornered off with road closed signs, this area served as our playground There we played hop- scotch, hide and seek, cricket, soccer and rugby.

The school was run under the auspices of the Union Congregational Churches and the principal and teachers all belonged to that domination.

The school was in the same street which we stayed, I would go to school early, and play and frolic on the school grounds.

I looked forward to school in the mornings and meet with my friends, they came from various race and cultural backgrounds in South End.

Discipline was the focus and the emphasis was on the 3 R's, Reading; Writing and Arithmetic. At an early stage you were inculcated with a strong work ethic and strive to do your best at all times. Moral education was given by the school through hymns, bible stories and religious instruction. The ethos of the school was "A sound body in a sound mind".

My school uniform was hand-me-downs from my elder brother, pants and shirts were made by my mother, a dress maker. My parents could not afford school shoes so I would go bare feet.

I was the second youngest, I had two brothers and two sisters. We were given chores before my mother left for work in the mornings, she worked as a domestic servant for a white family. She also took in washing from two white families who lived in the central part of town. We had the responsibility of collecting it and returning it washed and ironed.

My father worked as a waiter at a local country club. He worked long hours and would return late at night after a long day at work. My mother would dish up our food and place his in a colander on top of the prima stove. As children we were sorely tempted to eat the piece of meat and potato from his plate, on many occasions he would discipline us with his leather army belt. Although my father due his long working hours was for all intents and purposes an absent father, had a profound effect on me to learn a disciplined life. My mother through her hard work as a domestic, mother, wife and the added responsibilities had a tremendous impact on all facets of my life. She was a devout Christian and through her example taught us as children that we reach great heights in life with hard work.

We were very poor, but was able to cope with the demands of life by working as team. As children we were taught a independence and tolerance. My elder brothers helped to augment the family's income by working newspaper vendors. My responsibility was to by the groceries, meat and vegetables, at the cheapest prices. I had a tattered green bag which I tucked under my arm as walked the shops of South End to buy the groceries.

Our parents couldn't afford to give us pocket money, it was up to us children to find ways to make pocket money for our entertainment. I help my older brothers deliver newspapers, the income I made from that I used to go to the bioscope and for buying sweets. We left home at 4a.m to deliver the newspapers "the Herald" to the white residents in Summerstrand, Humewood and Millpark, Got home in time to go to school, I was very mischievous, I would sell the newspapers, but instead of declaring the money I would keep in and use it to purchase ice-cream at Chelsea Dairy, Twisted cones at Lee-Ching and Toffees at Damon. When I was found out I got one hell of a hiding from my father. Before you become a mason you have to work under someone is qualified. My brother worked as an apprenticeship mason at Evans Construction. Mr. Johns was Foreman. One of his responsibilities was to do the cooking in the house and the domestic chores. He prepared during the weekends curry bunnies which he sold to caddies at the whitey Walmer Country Club. He had a very dangerous job since he had to climb very high scaffolding. Once he fell and broke his leg and he was admitted to the hospital. We all South End Union church school which was run under the Union Church. The school was in the same street in which we stayed which meant it was easily accessible. I would go early to school to play with my friends in the school grounds. I looked forward to going to school and meeting up with my friends which came from various cultural groups. The school was also called the 'Blikskool' since the poorest children of the area attended the school. The schoolchildren wore hand-me-downs-, khaki pants which were made by the parents. We walked to school barefoot because our parents could not afford shoes. Our parents could not afford pocket money. We took a potato bag and walked through the streets of South End collecting bottles and bones. We exchanged this at FINRO Hardware adding stones to increase the weight of the bones. They never found that out.

Chapter 6
The Lonely Mind

Once upon a time long ago, more years than I care to remember I decided not to return to university to complete my teacher's diploma but rather to complete my B.Sc. Honours in Botany at the University of the Western Cape. I was refused admission due to my political past. I decided to teach and bank my salary in order to repay the government loan I had received in order to complete my degree. I got a teaching degree at my alma mater South End High School in January 1965. I was excited and looked forward to the challenge although my teaching roster was very loaded. For the standard sixes I had social studies and general science. I took the standard sevens for history and taught another class history in Afrikaans and then there were my standard nine classes. I taught physiology and hygiene. This was one of the main reasons which militated against me making a success of my teaching career. Many of the pupils were older than myself and I found myself teaching in the medium of Afrikaans even though I never had a teaching certificate. The students were difficult. I felt frustrated as if I could not get through to them. Of course I didn't realise I could not relate to them and they could not relate to me. For the large part they were undisciplined. Large classes made circumstances for effective teaching impossible. For the first three months I managed to cope however come to April I started to slow down. I could not concentrate on my lesson plans and found it easier to give up. I frequently fell into fits of depression and spells of self-pity. I found it difficult to teach. I was completely disinterested and demotivated. I found myself withdrawing from social interaction at school and at home. I left for school in the morning and stayed in the classroom for the rest of the school day. There was no discipline in the classes as I said before. This made things even tougher for me. I was disorganised. The pupils carried on acting out. They did just as they pleased. Pupils ran riot all over me, I virtually dragged myself through a school day. I had no assistance or support from my colleagues or people who I considered to be my friends. I also had no appetite and could not fall asleep at night. I was like a zombie from Hollywood B-movie dragging myself to school and home and back again. The doctor diagnosed me with having a vitamin deficiency. Anxiety overwhelmed me as I fell more and more behind with my lessons. I was overtaken by guilt of the injustice I was doing my pupils. I asked myself questions like who would be responsible if the pupils had to fail their examinations. Could I blame the principal, parents, learners or myself? I now felt like I was in a bottomless pit and in a dark tunnel. This was what always wavered on my mind those days. A feeling of gloom began to overwhelm me and suicide seemed to be the only way out. My thought process slowed down almost until it came to a standstill. My mind was completely clouded with negativity. After school I would spend the majority of my time in my bedroom. I vividly remember putting a plastic bag over my head. It burst before I suffocated. My mother was the only one who stood by me during this difficult time of my life. She prayed for me and saw that I had something to eat, had clean clothing. If that was hell what was to follow was even a greater hell. The viciousness of depression lifted and symptoms in direct contrast to the previous phase prevailed. I became talkative, loud, agitated. I walk around the whole school and the vicinity where I lived. I visited and spoke to people I never knew before. Within two weeks I spent all my savings which I religiously accumulated over a period of six months on useless items like antiques, liquor, old music records. Gifts were brought for people I met for the first time and I spent no time of the person. I did not sleep at night. I had no concern for my welfare. I did not listen to the people who had my best interests at heart. I could not bring myself to eat anything and walked long distances. Up streets and down streets. I decided to walk along the National Road to Cape Town. The road was pitch dark. This did not matter since I had a lot of energy. I got a lift in a furniture truck as far as Swellendam and then proceeded to the Meyer family in Bellville South. Two ministers of the United Congregational Church had me admitted as a voluntary patient at the Valkenburg Psychiatric Hospital in Pinelands Cape Town. For the first time I realised that I was in a mental institution when on admission I was given a polo jersey, khaki shorts and a pair of sandals. I was placed in a locked up ward. The patients came from all walks of life and suffered from all forms of mental illness. I was not diagnosed with any mental illness however I was not released from the locked up ward. However I must admit that it was therapeutic to be among other mentally ill sufferers. However I missed Port Elizabeth and my family. After a month at Valkenburg Psychiatric Hospital I took my leave to the medical school at Groote Schuur where I wanted to be in the first place. I then meandered through District Six where I found families dismantling their homes and belongings as a result of the forced removals of 1965.These residents were being moved to the Cape Flats and areas like Mitchell's Plan, Lavenderhill. These are now the centres of gang warfare. I sought help from the social worker at Groote Schuur Hospital. They supplied me with cigarettes, pocket money, and a third class railways ticket to Port Elizabeth. On the train I discovered that I had left the ticket in the jacket I had loaned while in Cape Town. Therefore I had no ticket on the train with the result that the guard and the policeman wanted to put me off the train at the next station. They were reluctant to believe my explanation. When reaching Port Elizabeth they handed me over to the police where I had to sign an undertaking that I would pay the cost of the ticket as I began teaching again.

The manic episode in Kimberly

My services had terminated at the South End High School. In January 1966 I was offered a temporary post

High School in Square Hill Park in Kimberly. I made a grave mistake by not checking on my medication. There was no psychiatrist or doctor who could describe mood stabilising drugs. I arrived in Kimberly on the 1st of February. The first month went okay. I gave my lessons clearly and meaningfully then all hell broke loose. I experienced a major episode of mania. I could not stop myself from making grave errors in judgement. I took myself to teach on a Saturday morning. During which time I consumed excessive amounts of whisky and milk. I spend long hours at school disturbing other teachers in the classrooms. I was creating complete mayhem in the school. I was not prepared to listen to the advice of well-meaning individuals. I also took to drinking alcohol. My meagre salary militating it becoming an uncomfortable habit. I spent a daily visit to the Kemo Hotel. I shudder to reflect on my manic state during the inter-Provincial swimming tournament of the Swimming Federation of South Africa. All the provinces from all over South Africa took part. I took charge of all the arrangements of the tournament, although I had no knowledge of competitive swimming. It was a disaster from the start. Without anybody's permission I appointed myself the manager of the Griqua Team. This was extremely embarrassing to the rest of the Griqua officials. I placed myself in charge of the bus which was going to transport teams and officials to a holiday resort along the Vaal River called

I in my pants and vest was trying to swim in the baby pool much to the amusement of the crowd.

I visited a family in Kimberly and was attracted by their son's toy gun which resembled a real gun. I went around the area and scared people as if it was a real gun. People began to avoid me as the stigma of mental illness was pronounced. I spent a night with a homosexual.

In April 1966 I returned to Port Elizabeth. My mania had abated and I obtained a temporary teaching post at the Gelvandale Secondary School. It was located in Helenvale which was a sub economic area and was established as a result of the slum clearance scheme of the municipality and the government

The area was soon overcrowded three primary and one secondary school was built in the space of three years

Ten people had to use one outside toilet. The streets were scattered with litter and dirt. The pupils came mainly barefoot to school and without any lunch. My class had more than 60 children. There were insufficient desks and writing materials. These circumstances made my teaching days in the beginning difficult, sad and depressing.

I had taken Zoology as one of my degree subjects. I collected stray cats. I placed one on a glass sheet which I covered with a bell jar and placed chloroform on wadding and placed it under the bell jar. I had underestimated the strength of the drugged cat.

In November 1966, the year mark for General Science and Social Studies had to be prepared for moderation by the Inspector of Education. At that time I fell into another deep episode. I slowed down, demotivated to do the simplest of tasks. I felt deep exhaustive depression. In the absence of the principal the deputy showed no sympathy for my depression. The day before the Inspector arrived my work was not yet complete yet the Inspector Mr Swanepoel ordered me to leave the school immediately despite the explanation of my depression. Fortunately for me the principal had just arrived from Cape Town. He assessed the situation, told me to see a doctor and to return to teaching when I felt well again. As I left the school to board the bus I was overwhelmed by suicidal thoughts. I had a strong desire for the bus to crash. This was not to be. I was alone at home and decided to take an overdose of tablets. It turned out to have the opposite effect. It didn't even make me drowsy or sleepy. The tablets that I did take turned out to be too few to have a serious effect. I got to the Port Elizabeth Mental Health Society where I received help.

Suicide was uppermost in my mind to the extent that I was continually thinking about taking an overdose of tablets. Fortunately my mother's early return from work removed these negative thoughts from my mind.

I was taken to the humble offices of the Port Elizabeth Mental Health Society in Brassell Street in North End where the social workers in particular Jan Hollingshead spent almost three hours of therapy with me so I could realise that suicide was not the only way out in a crisis situation. The next day I had an appointment with the psychiatrist in the outpatient department of the Livingstone hospital. He diagnosed me with manic depression also known as bipolar mood disorder. The seriousness of my condition necessitated five sessions of electroconvulsive therapy. A white patch had to be applied to both sides of my head which got me the nickname of the Western actor Jack Palance. I felt very sore and hurt when I heard these remarks made by people who I thought were my friends. I was also very young. I had never heard of electroconvulsive therapy before.

Since I was not aware of what it was I was very apprehensive at every occasion when I had to receive the treatment. However the white doctor who was in his fifties explained to me that the seriousness of my major depressive episode necessitated this treatment. He also gave me the assurance that the treatment wasn't a guarantee that I was to recover. I didn't know what the hell was going on the day I left the hospital that day. I was twenty years old.

In 1974 I won a scholarship by the British Council to complete a study of the mentally and physically handicapped in England and Wales and implement it in the position in South Africa. It was a very valuable scholarship since it covered a return plane ticket, tuition fees, books, warm clothing and even a maintenance grant. I was very happy, excited and content to undertake the scholarship and complete the relevant study. All went well up to the Christmas recess when the English students went home for the holidays. I with my friend, Jones Mceke and other African students was left behind to make provision for ourselves. I took the opportunity to organise a trip via Cosmos travel agency to visit five or six of the European countries. This was a dream come true for me since I visited Brussels in Belgium, Cologne and Frankfurt in Germany, Florence, the Vatican, Rome, Paris and then back via Dover. One of the most remarkable incidents happened to me at the customs at Dover. I was placed in a room with my luggage where I was asked to open my cases so that the customs officials could search my clothing. They also asked me a number of questions concerning my place of origin, why I had come to London and when I was going to return to South Africa again. After about two hours I was allowed to go. I then bordered the train to Euston Station which was not far from the residence. I was very, very down, depressed and sad at the happening at Dover. And I just wanted to go home to South Africa, however my friend

Jones was waiting for me. He helped me with my luggage and got me to my room. I realised that a major episode of depression was on its way. I had no appetite. I was exhaustibly tired. I couldn't fall asleep and I didn't know what to do because just before I left a young black student from Kenya who was manic depressive was sent home without getting suitable treatment. I thought that the same fate would face me. I couldn't get up out of bed in the morning. And I only responded to persistent knocking of my friend Jones. He got me out of bed. He saw to it that I got dressed and washed and virtually forced me to go to a nearby restaurant where I could enjoy some breakfast. I felt much better after that but not good enough. He took me back to my room where he sorted my clothing and placed the dirty clothing in a bag and took me to a Laundromat where he saw to it that I washed my clothing. Jones saved me. I wouldn't be sitting where I am today, surrounded by a loving and supportive family and my first grandchild, my son's son if it wasn't for Jones Mceke. Jones not only saw to my physical needs but was always encouraging and motivating me to allow the dark clouds of negativity and depression to lift. Fortunately when the university reopened I felt much better and could take my meals in the canteen and attend lectures as well as school visit in the English countryside. I must emphasise that I really enjoyed the greenery of the countryside. I will never forget my trip from London to Glasgow on the Express that travelled from the one end of England to the rest of Glasgow in Scotland. For the first time I could appreciate where English literary figures and poets could get their inspiration.

This was the most difficult phase of my life. I did not envisage the hell of a bipolar mood disorder. I was not in a position to prepare myself for the hell which was going to confront me

These initial experiences were primarily responsible for motivating me to write this book.

On arriving back in Port Elizabeth, I was successful in obtaining a temporary teaching post, but I certainly did not want to be a teacher. Deep down I had a yearning to be with my incarcerated comrades on Robben Island. I started to teach in January 1964 at my alma mater, South End High School. It was a disaster from the onset, not only was I too young at age 20 years, but I was not qualified to teach most of the subjects that were allocated to me. Many of the pupils were older than myself and I was required to teach subjects like History, Geography and Social Studies in the medium of Afrikaans. The fact that I only had an academic qualification, namely a B.Sc. Degree and lack of a professional teaching diploma militated against me making a success of teaching. This was exacerbated by the fact that I did not get much support from the other teachers on the staff.

I struggled desperately, but soon fell into a state of deep depression in April of that year. I started to withdraw from contact both in and outside school. Remaining in my room, refusing to see or speak to anyone, I lost my appetite, hardly slept, was tearful, listless and exhausted. I walked up and down in my room at home and at school. Teaching became extremely difficult as my thought processes slowed down. Discipline in the classroom became non-existent with the children doing as they please. As mentioned previously I had received no support from any of the other teachers.

By May 1965 I had all the symptoms of deep depression, but the tragedy was that no one at school, home or in the community realized that I was seriously ill. For five months I operated like a zombie, dragging myself to school in the morning, agonizing through the school day and then home again. It was a vicious circle, which was interrupted by weekends and school holidays, which I spent indoors in complete isolation. The tunnel was dark; yes very dark indeed.

With the arrival of winter in June 1965, suicidal thoughts dominated my thinking. I felt that suicide was the only way out of what was to me a hopeless situation. However the support and particularly the prayers of my mother prevented me from taking my own life.

My state of limbo continued until September 1965 when my mother got me to the humble offices of the Port Elizabeth Mental Health Society. The social workers of the society got me an appointment to see a state psychiatrist who referred me to the psychiatric department of the Livingstone Hospital in Port Elizabeth. I was placed on medication and received my first of many series of electro-convulsive therapy (etc), which proved to be ineffective. With the support of the social workers of the Port Elizabeth Mental Health Society and medication, the deep depression slowly began to lift. But the long period of the episode of deep depression had taken its toll.

The heavy feeling of depression began to lift with the concomitant relieve. The mood of darkness which made me think that suicide was the only solution was lifting and this brought me new hope to my life. This feeling only was a temporary flame of mind.

Just when I thought I was over the worst, another hell struck me. I went into a state of hell called mania.

The elation was a state directly opposite to the deep depression I had just come out of and I was completely out of control. I walked around aimlessly visiting unknown places and speaking to people I never usually spoke to. This happened at all hours of the day as I slept only for a few hours at night if at all.

I had an uncontrollable amount of energy, and felt restless all the time with no direction in anything I would do. No one could control me, not even my mother. One of the most tragic happenings of this phase of my illness was my uncontrollable spending of money. All the money I had so religiously saved during the year was spend in the matter of weeks on unnecessary items such as liquor, records, antiques an unnecessary clothing. It was through the grace of God that I did not bring about irreparable physical harm to myself or anybody else.

In the classes, to whom I had barely taught I was talkative. I now realize with hindsight that I spoke incoherently, disjointedly and my behaviour was bizarre and completely out of character.

I spoke excessively loud and much of which I conveyed in the classroom was totally irrelevant. My behaviour come under the attention of the headmaster who was at sea to understand what was the matter.
My behaviour in staff meetings was also a loud and incoherent contribution. It was a far cry from the virtual trance during the episode of depression. My condition was exacerbated by the lack of concern and support of my colleagues.

It took the headmaster some time before he could convince me to leave the school premises and take sick leave for an indefinite period. I was reluctant to accede to his request.

Just like with depression none of the local General Practitioners could diagnose my condition.

My irrational and bizarre behaviour caused much consternation to my family. It was particularly difficult on my sister who attended the same school I was teaching at. She had to endure the taunts of fellow-pupils and repulsive stigmatization from neighbours.

My mother who was a strong hearted individual had the necessary guts to bring my under a semblance of control.

I lived in a very close community, where everyone knew his neighbour. It was easy for my depression and later the manic state became common knowledge.

This would play a significant role on the stigma of bipolar mood disturbance would have on me in subsequent years.

My behaviour which went hand in hand with an uncontrollable amount of energy and feeling restless all the time with no direction in anything I would do.

Since the Port Elizabeth Mental Health Society (PEMHS) played such a significant role in the stability of my manic episode, it is necessary for me to narrate some of the work of the Port Elizabeth Mental Health Society.

Due to the system of racial separation the disadvantaged communities were provided with inadequate mental health facilities.

The aforementioned included psychiatric hospitals and clinics that were grossly understaffed and under equipped.

Patients who suffered from a mental disability like bipolar mood disorder were in the main locked up in what were called mental hospitals which were dilapidated buildings. These mentally ill patients were treated like animals with the prognosis being virtually zero. That would have been my fate, if I did not have the PEMHS intervening on my behalf. During the 1960's psychiatric facilities and treatment for disadvantaged patients were provided by the Port Elizabeth Mental Health Society. This was run mainly by volunteers and a minimal subsidy by the State. Community funds were utilized to pay for the rental of the buildings and to pay for transport costs of the patients and their families who were residents in distant localities.
If it was not for the dedicated staff of the PEMHS I would have come just another statistic in a dilapidated psychiatric enclave far away from my family and effective mediation and treatment.

However I must point out that no effective mood stabilizer and major tranquilisers were available to abate the mania.

It was only through the consistency, kindness, patience and love of the staff of the PEMHS that I persevered to gradually control my disturb mood disorder.

Other mentally ill patients were not so fortunate. During the 1960's -1980's any member of the disadvantaged mentally ill and psychological were handcuffed, placed in a straightjacket and locked up in the nearest police cells. The following day they would be transported to a makeshift psychiatric hospital. Here a cruel fate awaited them.

Cheaper medication which had a high toxic level which I was dispensed with had concomitantly horrendous side effects which made recovery difficult and unpleasant.

As unpleasant as this was, I had to tolerate the grave injustice of an Apartheid Health System.

During those difficult years organizations like the PEMHS played a key role in fighting the inequalities in the Mental Health Field.

At this I need to point out that the Society arranged that I saw a psychiatrist on a regular basis, got my monthly supply of medication and the social workers were always available to play the role of not only social worker, but also of psychologist, nurse and friend.

I was deeply honoured when I was appointed on the executive of PEMHS in 1984 and appointed an Honorary Life Member of the Society in 1999.

Chapter 7
Sixteen Words, the School Bell Tolls

My parents never taught me about how to go about making friends for life. Life overwhelmed me as a child. It overwhelmed me again as a young, inexperienced teacher, as a suitor wooing the young woman who was to become my future wife, that bride in her wedding lace and that virginal bride. And then it overwhelmed me again as a married man, as a father with three small children who looked up to me. I had to play mentor and role model. Depression is a malevolent story meant for grownups. The order of life there is somehow flawed. You ask yourself whatever happened to the routine of it all. There is no arrangement in the vase. You want to pick it up and hurl it across the room because that is what women do. Standing still they will compose themselves amongst the shitty life of the bits and pieces of it all or they will collapse. And they will come to the realisation that they will have to get the broom and sweep up this mess. Men can't do that. Men can't become emotional. They just don't have that kind of mentality. They don't have it within them unless they are alcoholics. Now there's romanticism for you. Women on the other hand. Well they become emotional at that moment. They cannot find the correct expression to wear on their faces.

All they can do is perhaps to mess up their hair and makeup. All they can do is wear their lipstick on their teeth, burst into tears and wait for someone to show up and rescue them. They do not know the proper way of how to go about to address madness. The instant they become spontaneously overwhelmed in the moment they reveal the source of their vulnerability.

Sometimes a man can wish he can be like a woman. That he can be an open book to the world. That he can have that sweet face. Man is driven to be physical when he is enraged. That is his nature. He lives and breathes by instinct. He follows through with that impulse. He can't waste his thoughts, time and energy infinitely like a woman on self-pity. Women truly loathe themselves. They think they can only be respected if they are perfectly put together inside and out. They relish the jealousy of other women their age. They want to be seen as beautiful first. They don't really care about having those brains, having that intelligence if they haven't had a father or a mother figure to instill that, the origins, the structures in them from a young age. They leave it to men to be confident leaders.

And when women have a mental sickness, when women are haunted by hallucinatory apparitions it is said in polite company that they are troubled. Perhaps talk will go as far as to say that they are deeply troubled. With men it is different. He becomes a drooling figure of fun. He becomes a clown with floppy shoes that are much too big for him to walk around in and behind his painted smile and dammit his jokes really aren't that funny. In the hospital you think that every hour is your last. I was a sportsman when I was younger although you wouldn't say it now. You wouldn't say it because I have belly fat. I have a stomach that hangs over my pants. You would think it is maybe because I drink too much beer over the weekends or have that single malt whisky hidden in the bottom draw and indulge in watching sport on the television. I do indulge in too much greasy, fatty food which I probably shouldn't. But that is what this disease can do to you. Turn your brains into a fatty soup. Make you feel ecstatic at meal times. Sometimes it can make you feel dead inside. Sometimes you feel as if the fabric of your skin is illuminated. As if it is dazzling. I don't long for a cigarette. I gave up smoking years ago before my children were born.

And I stuck to it in a way that I never thought was possible. There's a brightness around me sometimes. I know I am going under that bridge again and when that depression returns I do sometimes feel a terror inside. A terror that I am never going to really come all the way back. I am never going to be the same husband and father to my children. The depression and I have become inseparable from each other. I can't bring myself to cut the umbilical cord between us. I can't completely believe that I am the one that nurtures and gives the melancholia life. The diagnosis is night. I look at my wife. In all her femininity, the folds of her dress as she walks brushing against her ankles, her painful toes in her heels, I realise that she is physically stronger than me because she fights the depression within her. Whenever she feels it coming upon her she can counterattack it. She is the leader while I become diminished in her sight. A diminishment I cannot erase no matter how hard I try in my recovery period at home after I return from hospital life. It is another world, another country. Novel landscapes that I must get used to again and again and again. Children running under foot. Children are growing older. Going home to a house where you hear children's laughter takes getting me a while to get used to.

She needed to be loved, embraced and accepted by a man of all things in this world. And it had to be a beautiful man. All of those holier than thou sacred rituals that spelled personal success at the end of the rites of passage into young adulthood. As a father I knew she wanted and needed all of those rituals religiously. But she was already lost. She needed a lighthouse. She didn't know it but she needed one. I wanted to ask her. I had questions. Do you want a man who is in love with his own voice? Do you want a man who is not going to listen to you? A man who is not a warm and sincere listener? Or do you want to live with a man who wants his ego stroked all day and all night? For they are all out there to be embraced by a young woman who has little or no self-esteem or worth. And what do you think of a man who causes an injury to another man thinking very little or nothing about it? Who does not think of sparing his enemy that slight or that humiliation? What do you think of a woman who injures another woman? Man against woman. Woman against man. All the time causing an injury. And I think that what I am touching is pure art because all art is borne of pain and injury. I think of my daughter, the child who will forever be caught in the middle for the rest of her life.

She is leaving me behind in the dust with those imaginary shadows. Leaving me behind with those ghosts. I wanted to tell her all of the things even though I knew my warning would fall on deaf ears. She didn't want to be my accomplice. She didn't want to take up her place in a line of a succession of feminists. Standing in line was not meant for a girl like her. A young lady who had goals and dreams, norms and values and who had not dreamt of suicide a day in her life like her older sister had. Her older sister who becomes a sullen teenager who does not like the way the hairdresser cuts her hair and who complains about everything. Her mother's erratic behaviour, her mother's quaint sayings that were like small explosions going off, the way she cooks and the preparation that goes into her food. My daughters, my daughters, my daughters. I could not protect them forever. And I was slow to come to that realisation. Slower to come to accept. I had to learn to accept it. My daughters were like weeping willows. At night I would creep into their bedrooms and watch them sleep. Watch them inhale and exhale in all their innocence of that dark and cruel world outside the doors of this house.

This house that I had built. On the beach they had the song of willows in the hair and when they cried out my name I felt something twist inside my heart. Was it pain? Was it something that had the great depths of beauty? It made me feel like a wreck. A beautiful design by seawaters wreck with that had those symmetries. I wondered if they would carry all the symbolic treasures of their childhood into young adulthood with them. The moon of their childhood. Their sunburnt legs licked by wind and the elements. And I counted the days of how soon they would find the suffering in their exciting childhood. When the children weren't in the house. When they were at Speech and Drama or a swimming lesson or an extra class to catch up on English or Mathematics I would walk through all the rooms in the house. It was as if they had left an imprint of their physical bodies and their laughter behind and somehow it seemed to mask the anguish and the pain I felt of the fact that one day soon I would have to let them go. I would have to surrender them to the unknown, to the wilderness, to that wasteland that was both reality and the universe and they would have to figure out for themselves what a metaphysical survival would mean to them.

Their fingerprints were there even though I could not see them against the walls of the interiors of the house. Adults pride themselves on the gift of investing in themselves, perfecting themselves but not acquiring the gift of love. Love is more like a holiday. Easter. Christmas. Most if they're lucky think it is merely a temporary frame. A flame. That waterfall. That teardrop. After hospital life I soon got over the shock of standing still, waiting and recovering. After all insanity was just a relapse into an otherworldly experience and the wonderful thing about life is that we are all searching for a metaphysical survival after surviving a traumatic experience. That storm that leaves us bloodied, feeling pins and needles in our hands, feeling desolate and alone with our hearts filled with despair at the thought of what will happen next. Survival will always be there making an honest living. There will always be a cave out there for sanctuary. But what am I really afraid of? Sometimes I fear I am missing a part of myself because of this mental sickness. That I am the screaming man. That the big, bad wolf has finally got hold of me with its mouth and its crazy jaws. I had those women on my arm in youth. I had been in love numerous times because that is sometimes the nature of the illness.

I was like ordinary people. I was afraid of debit. I bought it on credit. I was lonely.

In the ward at that posh clinic you went to for a week you find yourself feeling flat. You also find that you need to write and the words pour out of you like wine. You can taste its sweetness. You find that you are thirsty all the time. And everyone, every single person there becomes a sexual object to you. You no longer see the individual behind the person. If people could read your mind, could read your thoughts they would see an arrogant bastard who knew everything there was to know about the world of the egotistical alpha male and the bewilderment of craziness and acting crazily, talking crazy, walking around wounded and scarred for life by the images of religion. The purification rituals of religion. You think of the church, of your faith as your second home, your second family. You need water. You need to drink. You need to empty this self-pity out of you. It feels liquid (of course it's liquid) this weight of water filling up your chest. Manoeuvring its way to your heart and finding its way to your platelets and your brain.

Nobody tells you how to go about making friends for life when you are mentally ill. When you are forever carrying around this sickness within your heart. Jealousy is something else. It is one of the hardest things in this world to let go of. It is just supposed to happen as naturally as cold weather and snow in winter. Snow spreads out in a wild field or fields filled with hay in summertime. Poppies heads screaming to be heard. Screaming red. Signaling an emergency service. When you are a child, nobody tells you of the pressures of an adult life.

You find that you keep on asking yourself if this is a story for grownups because children will pick up on the awareness of illness, on the evils of this world. That exists because of the nature of man and frustration. Are you missing a part of yourself because you are no longer in love with the world or that you have come to the realisation that it is no longer in love with you? What has happened to you being in high spirits, being the life of the party? What has happened to your soul? It has turned into soup. It has turned dark out even though you can still feel the brightness of the day, the texture of the sun like the song says. I am afraid of sadness. The sameness. I am afraid of suffering and of the days that will come when I will no longer suffer. I do not reach for my wife anymore in the dark. It is no longer strange to me to find myself alone at night although I can still hear her breathing. I no longer feel the warmth of her body next to mine. But the doctors do not speak of this to you. They do not speak of the consequences and the challenges that you will have to face up to come hell or high water. Perhaps I think they might be too embarrassed to be open and honest with you. My wife and I, well we have become strangers to one another overnight. She no longer cooks for me.

Everything has become too much for her and I think it has a lot to do with me. It is my fault. Everything is my fault. Blame me. Blame me for the separation. Blame me for the fact that we were nearly divorced when our youngest was on the brink of becoming a teen-ager. Of course there are days when I feel I am missing a part of myself because it feels as if I am no longer in love. That I haven't got that woman on my arm anymore or in my arms at night. There are times that I am inclined to think that I am a victim and that I am not a survivor because that is the nature of illness. Having a disease or any kind of sickness will do that to you. I am the screaming man.

Chapter 8
University College of the Western Cape (1962 - 1964)

The university buildings consisted of a number of prefabricated classrooms of an old primary school, which were converted to lecture rooms, laboratories, library and the like.

The science buildings were in the process of being built and they were 3 kilometres on the road from Bellville South. Although the authorities had promised a bus service, there was no such service when the university opened for the academic year. So that morning when the university opened, 250 science students found themselves walking along the dusty road to the building site of the science building.

A few laboratories and lecture rooms were just about completed, but the whole scene was sand, sand and more sand, with scaffolding everywhere and workers milling around. I was completely devastated on discovering that most of the lectures were being given in the medium of Afrikaans. Science subjects like Zoology, Physics, Chemistry and Botany are difficult, but when given in the medium of Afrikaans, it becomes a nearly impossible task.

The whole university was Afrikaans orientated and no provision was made for students who were English speaking. However, the Afrikaans-speaking students also had a distinct disadvantage since there were no science textbooks available in the Afrikaans medium. The best we could do was to consult senior students who had already gone through the experience. They advised us that we should not discontinue our studies, but to knuckle down to some serious translation of the notes, consulting textbooks and assisting each other as far as possible.

We were also confronted with mainly under-qualified and inexperienced lecturers. To our dismay we discovered that the situation was not much better in the arts department that still operated from the ex-primary school in Bellville South. During the lunch break.

We discovered there was no cafeteria or tuck shop; therefore we joined the labourers who operated an iron through with ice and cold drinks. We lay on the sand and had our lunch. The situation was discussed and we were completely devastated when it was discovered that there was no one to address the serious state of affairs. Here was a case of the taxpayers' money being used to further a philosophy of apartheid in all its 'nakedness'.

These conditions at the university presented fertile ground for the development of political activity. Such a political group had its origin at my place of residence in Lloyd Street in Bellville South. The political program helped to appease our frustrations as young black students at a tribal university. This was like "manna from heaven" because it gave us some kind of rationale, some structure in which we could understand the realities of the situation we found ourselves in.

Conditions deteriorated daily and many students found it difficult to cope. Human potential was wasted tragically, because they had not been given a change. Certainly if they had to have a separate university for Coloureds then at least they could have seen to a basic infrastructure such as proper laboratories, canteen facilities, properly equipped library, suitably qualified lecturers who were fully bilingual, and so on.

These early years of the 60's were politically turbulent because it was at this time that the massacre at Sharpeville took place when 69 people were shot and killed. The whole scenario in the country was desperate and tragic. Blacks on the whole looked at the horror and brutality of Sharpeville as enough reason to reject the apartheid regime in toto. This in microcosm was the feeling of the students at the University College of the Western Cape.

So this was the early breeding ground of the armed struggle, which was subsequently chosen by the liberatory forces as the only salvation in fighting the National Government.

The university authorities took tough steps against any criticism voiced by the student body against the appalling conditions at the university. This did not prevent student activists from being involved in liberatory politics. To escape the attention of the security police, regular trips were organized to Table Mountain where the discussion of deep political issues took place.

I left home in the mornings at 7 o'clock and only returned at around six in the evening with no proper midday meal, political debates, translating notes of the day, completing tutorials meant working until the early hours of the morning. It was hard work and at times frustrating, but I realised that I would only be successful if I worked extremely hard. Most of the science students could not keep up with the pace of the work, and gradually spent less time with their books and more time in the social scene. I could see the signs of catastrophic happenings for the frustrated students as time progressed.

It is important for the reader to be made aware of what was called the duty performance system (D.P System) This system involved the student obtaining at least 40% in test June/September test and other tests during the year before you were allowed entrance to the final examination. Other universities like the

University of Cape Town also used the system, but their D.P. Equivalent was 25%. In my own case, having had to adapt to the Afrikaans, and due to the lack of proper facilities, together with the attitude of some of the lecturers, placed me in a serious dilemma. Leading up to the September examination I had to obtain more than 60% in most of my subjects in order to obtain the required D.P.'s.

Because most of the students had performed poorly in the work earlier in the year, it meant they had to obtain very high marks in order to obtain the required D.P. Most science students with the September examination looming, began to lose interest in the academic program as they gave up all hope of obtaining the required D.P.'s

Students were not against a D.P. System, but they objected to the rigid way in which it was implemented by the university authorities. The authorities refused to address the problems with them. Of the approximate 250 students who started the course, there were fewer than a hundred who were still attending lectures. Students realised that the system, as well as other circumstances which prevailed at the university, was a deliberate attempt by the Nationalist Government to deny black students the right to higher education particularly in the field of science. They were making sure that black students were not going to become scientists such as physicists and chemists.

One of the statistics that will remain in my mind is that of the chemistry class, which started as a class of 200; only 25 obtained D.P. 's and only 7 ultimately passed the final examination. For the first time I saw students crying on D.P. day when they realized that their studies were officially over without being allowed to write an examination. They had failed without being given a chance. When students questioned the conditions at university, they were told that they should not involve themselves in politics. We were in contact with other tribal universities and discovered that similar conditions prevailed on these campuses. I was very fortunate to obtain D.P. 's in all my subjects, but entered the examination period with trepidation, fearing the possibility of victimisation. I worked very hard and was one of the fortunate few who managed to pass all my subjects.

I had just completed my Masters of Education Degree and registered for the Doctor of Philosophy in 1984 when the position of Headmaster at Gelvandale High School became vacant.

Since I had been in the position of Deputy Principal of the school for the past five years, it was felt by the fellow educators and parents that I would be the most suitable candidate as headmaster.

However students felt that someone else should be appointed because I suffered from bipolar mood disorder.

The Educational Department appointed an outside person as headmaster. This had disastrous results for the school with educators, parents and pupils coming out in protest.

I personally felt that I had the qualifications, experience as well as my disorder was stable, to fulfill the position. I was hurt by the stigmatization; I had to bear it from various quarters including the Educational Department.

In April 1984 the School Committee (a body of elected parents) unanimously appointed me as headmaster of Gelvandale High School. This was one of the proudest moments in my teaching career, and as a sufferer of a bipolar mood disorder.

The school was a comprehensive school with 1250 pupils, 67 educators, a hostel and an ancillary staff of 30. It was indeed a great challenge since the school served a predominantly sub economic area.

I had got into a regular pattern of walking, swimming and exercising. These activities were enhanced by regular antidepressants antipsychotic and sleeping medication which made me reach a stable balance of my mood disorder.

My main aim was to knit the school family (pupils, parents and community into a coherent whole).

The period from 1984 was characterized by black pupil awareness of Apartheid, which resulted in intermittent school boycotts and stay-always. At the same time as running the school, I had to meet deadlines such as preparatory work for the Professor promoting my doctoral studies. I had to travel extensively to collect archival material from various libraries in Pietermaritzburg, Durban, Cape Town and Johannesburg.

This was a very expensive exercise, and with the absence of bursaries it was draining my resources. However I got a great deal of satisfaction from the turbulent periods as Headmaster as well as my doctoral research.

To date and with hindsight I do not know where I got the energy to meet the demands of such a busy schedule which included the position of husband and father of three children.

The school program progressed well although it had to be administered with inferior equipment and a dire shortage of sports, science and practical materials.

Throughout my period of Headmastership I experienced taunting and stigmatization. I worked very hard to overcome this state of affairs and did not allow it to affect the stressors which could cause me depression or mania.

The matriculation results, which was the barometer of the success of the school, was always above the average throughout the 10 years as Headmaster. (1984-1994).

After a really challenging period of doctoral studies at Rhodes University my hard work and perseverance played off. I finally graduated in 1989 with a PhD degree in Education.
(For a fuller account-see chapter)

Throughout the 10 years studying at Rhodes University and being Headmaster, I experience periodic spells of mood swings. I must state that the episodes never disrupted my studies or work as an educationalist.

Throughout this period I paid my monthly visits to the Port Elizabeth Mental Health Society. Here I obtained my monthly supply of medication. Also a quarterly basis saw the psychiatrist and received valuable psychotherapy from the social worker.

If it was not for the support I received from social workers Jan Hollingshead, Mrs. Levenstein and Mrs. Atwell I would not have been a success in the years 1980 - 1994.

On the advice of my psychiatrist I was admitted to the Elizabeth Donkin State Psychiatric Hospital, a hospital which was regarded in a poor light by the community of Port Elizabeth. But I had no choice, I had no medical aid funds and with a state pension I could not afford a private hospital.

The physical comfort at Elizabeth Donkin was very inferior to that which existed at Hunters Craig. My first impression of ward (R) was that of a dark garret out of Charles Dickens' "A Tale of Two Cities". On the stoep, there were chairs from which the stuffing had been horribly exposed and the sitting place was a large gaping hole.

I was received into an open office where nurses, social workers, nursing aids, psychologists, and doctors shared a common office space. The nurse who admitted me had the side of her face on the table and in this awkward posture she proceeded to ask me the most intimate details of my life. This was a most distressing experience, after which I was taken to my room.

My room reminded me of the John Wayne westerns I saw as a youngster. Firstly the bed was very high from the ground. I could not imagine what would happen to me if I fell off during the night. There was a basin but no running water, and even if there were, it would not have helped because there was no outlet pipe and in any case there was no plug. With much anguish I decided to have a bath. When I got to the bathroom I discovered there was no plug for the bath or the basin next to the bath. On making enquiries I was told by the nurse on duty that plugs were not supplied because patients steal them. She suggested that I should get the top of a Cabana Juice bottle, wrap it in toilet paper and try since it was the standard method of how patients solved the problem. I was in a state of disillusionment, very anxious and strongly tempted to leave the hospital in my sick state and to go home where I knew I would become even sicker.

I went to supper a very worried man, but God had not forsaken me. Fellow sufferers rallied around me and gave me material and moral support. After supper a short prayer meeting was organized and it was with a greatly relieved mind that I went to sleep that night. I realised that although I was suffering from depression and that the circumstances at Elizabeth Donkin were difficult, with the help of other fellow depression sufferers I was going to survive.

Roll call was at 6 o'clock every morning, and this was done by the ringing of a bell. All patients' male and female had to make their way to the lounge where they had to be counted by the staff coming on duty. This usually took a few minutes which meant 26 patients had to get out of warm beds and assemble to be counted because it was an effort for the day nurses to go from room to room to count the patients. There might have been a lot of merit in such a system, but it was never explained to me in a rational and logical manner. However, the fact that I completely accepted a sense of camaraderie among them made me feel very content.

The ward was run by ordinary general practitioners that worked under the supervision of a specialist psychiatrist who was in attendance on a Tuesday. This delay made treatment very difficult. Since I had been on a myriad of antidepressants, which did not seem to help, I was discharged after five weeks without any medication. The psychologist told me that I had to learn to live without antidepressants. I was no better than 5 weeks ago when I had entered the hospital dispirited, despondent and devastated. With suicidal thoughts uppermost in my mind when I left the grounds of the Elizabeth Donkin Hospital. I felt that there had been a travesty of justice against me. However, God's miracles that had sustained me through very difficult times before, I believed would sustain me now.

After leaving Elizabeth Donkin I went to my own GP who consoled me by stating that although I had been on a number of antidepressants, he felt that it would do me no harm to go on S.R. Inhibitor type of antidepressant. It was going to be a long wait because it would take at least 3 weeks before any improvement would be apparent. I waited anxiously, but come the end of September there was no improvement in the state of my depression. The doctor gave it another month without success. In November in what I would call a last ditch stand; he placed me on mono amine oxidase-type of antidepressant

Chapter 9
Inspector of Education

When I returned to school it was in disarray and pupil was boycotting classes because of poor facilities and lack of equipment. Boycotts could still go, but what really infuriated me was when teachers decided to go on strike. I became totally disillusioned with the strike action and decided to apply for the post of Inspector of Education. Since the ANC and PAC had been unbanned and with a new government inevitable, I felt that because the different ethnic groups were going to be transformed into one department it would be an ideal position to be in for an educationalist. On 2 January 1994 I was officially appointed Inspector of Schools with 45 schools in the Eastern Cape under my jurisdiction.

In 1995 we were required to attend meetings in Port Elizabeth and Bisho to take part in discussions on different aspects of education in preparation towards one educational system. Members of all four the educational departments were involved in discussions which at times became heated. I then realized that the transformation to one educational system was going to be a daunting task. I was of the opinion that all South Africans had a role to play in the transformation process to a Non-Racial, No-Sexist, Democratic Educational System.

The past had to be seen in a constructive light; namely all the good in the education of the past needed to be evaluated with the future in mind. I got the impression that many of the younger educationalists felt that anything from the past needed to be discarded. I thought this would be a tremendous waste and was deeply distressed by the manner in which the deliberations of such an important facet of the new South Africa education went.

In March 1996 I started to spend less time at the office and spent more time at home. I could no longer get myself out of bed in the morning and I felt too tired to go to the office. My appetite disappeared, I felt listless and gradually withdrew into my room and I did not even want to answer the phone. I am of the opinion that the conditions at the office exacerbated my depression. Up to this stage the reader is aware that I had been on the receiving end of the unjust apartheid regime of the Nationalist Government. Since birth, through my youth, at university, moving as a result of the Group Areas from South End, having to resettle and start a new life. I had been fighting for one non-racial democratic system of education all my life; it was one of my greatest dreams to see it realised.

Here my dream had become a reality; so-called White, African, Coloured and Indian educationalists were at last together to participate in truly historical events to assist in the transformation process of one educational system. My bout of depression brought my participation in the process to an end. To me this was a very tragic occurrence as I felt I had still so much to contribute. This feeling of despondency made me feel even more depressed and my condition deteriorated even further. Even the worthwhile contributions I had made could not make me feel better.

I chaired a task group representing the whole of the Eastern Province and was concerned with all facets of special education. I presented detailed memoranda to the Provincial Education Department concerning all facets of the severely mentally handicapped child in the province. I participated in workshop, seminars, plenary sessions, and task groups on all aspects of education, which was working towards the transformation of a Non-Racial, Non-Sexist Democratic System of Education. With hindsight and in all humility I feel that I had made a contribution to education in apartheid South Africa as well as in the new South Africa.

The depression was not going to lift and I was never going to recover to return to the teaching profession, which I so dearly loved and served so diligently for 32 years. In December 1996 at the age of 53 I was medically boarded as a result of chronic clinical depression with limited financial resources since most of my benefits were utilized to subsidise my prolonged sick leave.

The cycle of depression was taking its course, no antidepressant could help, and no tranquilliser or sleeping tablet could bring relief. I was hospitalised on 1 July 1997 at Hunterscraig Psychiatric Hospital. I immediately felt relieved. It was good to talk and live with fellow depression sufferers. What was indeed very striking was that the patients came from across the spectrum of the new South Africa colour of a person's skin or social standing had no place here. We were all depression sufferers.

There were medical doctors, ministers of religion, nurses, social workers, policemen, warders, traffic officers, housewives, teenagers, drug addicts, alcoholics, pensioners, unemployed, retrenched, abused attempt suicidal cases and the like. The patients, some, who were very ill on admission, felt much better by being in the environment of other depression sufferers. A unique bond of love and camaraderie bonded them. Really those two weeks were emotionally the best I had experienced for the last two years.

I also spent two weeks at Howe Psychiatric Clinic where we were taught life skills such as time management, conflict management, communication skills, stress management, assertiveness training. However, at the end of this period, I was told that I had been discharged because my medical aid funds had been used up. In desperation I explained my position to the senior matron that I am allowed to negotiate with my medical aid for additional funds. She would not budge; all she could say was rules were rules. Afterwards I even promised to pay it out of my pension, but she was unrelenting. The deep depression was returning and the hard work over the last three weeks by psychologists, psychiatrists, occupational therapists, and other members of the multidisciplinary health team was for nothing.

Chapter 10
Playing at Politics

A week after the completion of the examination, my friend and I were approached about the recruitment into a subversive organization. The time that we were approached was during the period, which I just described, with students like myself being totally devastated psychologically by the apartheid university structure. I had experienced much hurt and also seen much hurt experienced by others. Thus it was not difficult to decide to become a member of a subversive organisation, although I realised the grave consequences of taking such action.

At the age of 18, I decided that the armed struggle was the only way in which the illegitimate regime of the National Party was going to bring the desired results in the struggle for liberation for all South Africans. The aim of the organization (called the National Liberation Front) was to work towards a non-racial, non-sexist democratic South Africa in which the rural poor and the interests of the workers would be the predominant feature. Its policy of non-collaboration was important since it was felt that no oppressed person should work the machinery of his own oppression.

To me as a student of the University College of the Western Cape in 1963, the principle of non-collaboration was extremely attractive because as a disenfranchised student at a tribal university I was forced to attend the university. I was not forced to promote the establishment of an SRC, to attend any functions of the university or to play sport under the banner. The state was powerful; it depended on the army, police, riot squads, security police, 90 and 180 days detention, solitary confinement, heavy prison sentences and states of emergency for long periods to keep a grip on the country. The reader must realise that these were very difficult times in South Africa. The apartheid regime of Verwoerd was at its strongest, the police force was vicious and the security police was well organized.

The major advantages of belonging to the National Liberation Front were that it made me mentally strong and brought much discipline into my life. We took part in all the activities of the cell we belonged to; however, in June 1964 disaster struck the organization. The police had infiltrated some of the cells of the organization and in this way placed all of us belonging to it, at risk. The security police started to arrest senior members and gradually we realised that all of us had to prepare ourselves to be arrested.

We all knew the danger of belonging to a subversive organisation and the consequences of our actions.

The Western Cape students were known to the special branch, but it was an arrangement between the state and the defense that the accused would make full disclosures on the mechanics of the organization providing the students of the University of the Western Cape were not arrested or called to be state witnesses. This was a wonderful gesture of comradeship for which I will always be grateful.

The trials of the state versus the National Liberation Front were set in the Cape Town Supreme Court in which 10 members of the organization were accused of high treason. In some miraculous manner I obtained D.P. 's in all my subjects. The reader must be made aware of the exceptional mental ability of the Western Cape students who were in the cell of the National Liberation Front. We had all passed our final examinations despite the trauma of the past months.

The potent force in my case was my belief in the Almighty God and the prayers of my mother. My mother was extremely proud her son passed and I was going back in 1964 to complete my B.Sc. Degree. The trial had in the meantime ended, the judge found all the accused guilty of sabotage and sentences from 7 to 10 years were passed on all the accused. So that brought to an end an era in the University of Western Cape Resistance Politics. It was a travesty of justice that the accused had to be incarcerated since no building was sabotaged; nobody was injured or killed. The judgement in the case was absolutely mind boggling, and it was with heavy hearts that we read the sentence in the newspaper.

I was much more careful now, but the work of political education at the Western Cape continued unabatedly. I was committed to spending more time completing my degree, but there were many issues, which still cropped up. We had influenced many students to resist the apartheid ethnic "Bush University" concept. The whole of 1964 was taken up by the aftermath of the trial and giving assistance to the families of those comrades who were incarcerated on Robben Island.

In 1964 I fulfilled the requirements for the B.Sc. degree. With a first class pass in Botany. I was determined not to complete my teacher's diploma, but decided to pay back the bursary/loan which had got me to the University of the Western Cape in the first place, to accumulate funds and then go back and do a B.Sc. (Hon) in Botany.

During my three years at the UWC, I had no depression or manic periods, which affected my studies or extra-curricular activities at the university. There were periods of despondency, discouragement and gloom, but it was not extreme in nature that drastically affected my activities. My political activities, particularly the subversive organization, the arrest of its members, and their subsequent court appearance, was very traumatic for me and affected me psychologically. How the Western Cape experience with all its concomitant stresses would affect me in later life will become clear to the reader as my story further unfolds.

Chapter 11
Consolidation of Teaching Career

At this time, I had much progress in the manner in which I was handling my mood swings. The daily exercising program as well as swimming three times a week had stood me in good stead. My attitude towards teaching was much more positive and was approached with confidence and enthusiasm. I was also on a potent daily dosage of psychotropic medication which assisted me to cope with the manic and depressive episodes of bipolar disorder.

Thus in 1970 I took the reluctant decision to do my Secondary Teacher's Diploma at the UWC. In February I started my course of study. On my arrival in Cape Town I immediately reported to the psychiatric outpatient clinic at Karl Bremer Hospital. I attended the clinic on a monthly basis and I also received my medication on a one-month basis.

The authorities had appointed fellow students to spy on me in and outside the university boundaries. They wanted to know what I was speaking about and whether I was trying to influence the other students politically. I was not discouraged by these puerile attempts at disturbing my peace of mind. Although I was not keen to become a teacher, I decided that I came to the university to study towards a Secondary Teacher's Diploma and that is what I was going to achieve.

The road ahead was very tough since most of the lectures and notes were in Afrikaans. A daily priority was to translate the notes and I somehow managed to cope with the work. At the end of the year I successfully completed the Secondary Teacher's Diploma. My depression was stable through the whole year and this contributed in no small way to my success. In January 1971 I immediately registered for the postgraduate Bachelor of Education degree through the University of South Africa. I completed the degree within the stipulated two years; with a distinction in philosophy of education.

In 1972 I received my first promotion in my career, namely that of senior secondary assistant. In 1973 I tried to register for a Master of Education degree at the local University of Port Elizabeth. I discussed my proposal with the senior lecturer in the faculty of education. He was very excited about my proposed field of research and we spent many hours discussing it. The lecturer Dr. Smith was more than satisfied and it also received favourable comments from the professor of the faculty. All that was left to do was to register so that I could immediately commence my research.

Then came the shock. The registrar in his reply to my application informed me that the university regretted that they could not accept me as a master's student because of the Separate University Act of 1960. It stipulates that all students must attend the university the government has set aside for that population group. Since I belong to the so-called "coloured" population group, I had to attend the University of the Western Cape in Cape Town. Although the University of Port Elizabeth had refused me permission to do the Master degree in education,
I had not felt discouraged.

106

The completion of the STD and B.Ed. gave me a sense of stability, confidence and motivation to succeed in teaching. I continued my walking, swimming and exercising.

I continued to see the social workers at the PEMHS. They rendered a multifaceted function in my treatment, which included valuable psychotherapy at least once a month when I collected my medication.

Chapter 12
Me, Jones and London Town

Ever since I got to know myself, it has been my desire to travel overseas, particularly to London. In 1973 I saw an advertisement in the local newspaper inviting applications from suitably qualified South African professionals to the British Council for an academic year of study at any British university.

At the same time the American consulate invited applications from suitably qualified South African graduates for postgraduate study at any American university. Both these scholarships were very attractive because they included a return air ticket, full tuition fees, full residential fees, a monthly stipend, and a book allowance, and in Britain an allowance was also made for warm clothing.

My reaction to them was an ambivalent one, on the one hand as a black in apartheid South Africans, I was so conditioned that I was strongly convinced that these scholarships were only meant for white South Africans. I did not know of any blacks that had won these scholarships, however my greatest fear was that the government would not grant me a passport due to my political activity. On the other hand if I won one of these scholarships it would really be a lifetime dream come true. I got the necessary application forms and dually went through what I regarded as the motions because I was still convinced that I stood no chance and my qualifications did not compare with that of whites from the university of Port Elizabeth and Rhodes.

I went for both interviews in Port Elizabeth; conducted by professors of education from the universities of Rhodes and Port Elizabeth. Both universities catered only for white students at that time. From the nature of the questions, I was more than ever convinced that they were going to select only whites for the scholarships. However the major problem remained the passport.

My first study option was a research course of study in science teaching at high school level and the second option was a research study on the mentally and physically handicapped child.

After many months of correspondence with the British Consulate in Cape Town and the American Embassy in Pretoria I received the following correspondence, which I regarded as the greatest and happiest news of my life. Firstly, the American consulate awarded me two options to do postgraduate study at American universities. They were met with the option of doing a master degree in educational psychology at Columbia University, New York stretching over 3 years or the opportunity of doing a doctoral program in educational psychology at Washington University, over a period of 3 to 5 years.

Secondly, the British Council offered me a year of postgraduate study on the mentally and physically handicapped at the prestigious Institute of Education of London University leading to the title of "Associate of the University's Institute of Education.

My application for a South African passport was also successful. Here I had two offers that I had only dreamt about not so long ago and I had to answer within 2 weeks. Being a manic depression sufferer, I accepted the offer to study at the University of London, because I would only then be away for 10 months since the academic year at English universities stretched from October 1974 to June 1975. I realised that if I became ill, I would rather spend 10 months in London than 3 to 5 years in the United States of America. The American consulate could not understand my refusal of their offer and subsequently contacted me on many occasions trying to change my decision. The University of London was my choice and I stood by it.

I left Johannesburg international airport on the 21st September 1974 on a British airways jumbo jet. What an experience that was. More excitement was to follow when the flight arrived at Nairobi airport, Kenya at midnight. Here we were allowed to disembark and enter the transit lounge while the plane was busy refueling. What excitement for a South African student to be in an African country even if only in the transit lounge. To see all the African curios, materials, flags and other indigenous paraphernalia was exciting beyond belief.

The plane arrived at Heathrow international airport, London early the next morning. I was met by British Council officials and transported to Victoria station then to Euston station to arrive at the St Adams hall of residence, Endsleigh Street, London WC! Where I was escorted to a single room. Here I was in a matter of only 18 hours from apartheid South Africa to the cosmopolitan city of London where the practice of apartheid was illegal. I cannot transcribe the euphoria I felt when I entered the lounge and bang in front of a television, the first one I had seen in my life because in 1974 television was unknown in South Africa?

I was alone in the lounge since I was one of the first students to arrive. The television was off and I stood transfixed in front of the big box not knowing what to do. My stupor was lifted with the entrance of a student from Ghana who after introducing himself switched on the television and asked me whether I wanted to watch BBC 1 or BBC 2. I told him I was from South Africa and this was the first time in my life I saw a television set. Let alone BBC 1 or BBC 2.

One of the most remarkable occurrences was to meet and stay with students from all over the world. These included countries like Ghana, Sierra Leone, Somalia, Kenya, Ethiopia, Tanzania, Zambia, Zimbabwe, Egypt, Algeria, Malaysia, Japan, Hong Kong, Indonesia, America, West Indies, Fiji, Argentina, Peru and the like. I bonded well with the overseas students and had a bosom friend, Jones Mceke, from Zambia who stood by me at all times.

After registration I joined a class which consisted of 7 English students who were all experienced teachers in schools for the handicapped in England, Scotland and Wales, 3 students from Hong Kong, Malaysia, Ghana and myself. While working towards our research we attended lectures on neuropsychological, child defects and handicaps. We also attended lectures, workshops and seminars on the psychological and educational aspects of the handicapped child. Weekly visits were organized to schools and colleges for handicapped children all over London and its surroundings.

All went very well, so well that over the Christmas recess of 1974 I went on a guided tour of Brussels in Belgium, Lucerne and Geneva in Switzerland, Florence, Venice and Pisa in Italy, Cologne and Frankfurt in Germany, Paris in France and back via Dover. At Dover the strangest incident happened to me. At customs I was taken to a small room where every piece of my luggage was searched and the customs officials interrogated me for almost 2 hours. It became apparent that they believed from my appearance that I came from one of the Arab countries and was carrying a false South African passport.

I was in a deranged and confused state as a result of the detention and interrogation; it reminded me of the trauma I had suffered at the hands of the security branch of the South African police during my activist years as a student at the UWC. Thus for the first time in Britain I felt I was back in apartheid South Africa. I am of the opinion that this was the major stress factor which precipitated my major depression attack in London in January 1975.

The PEMHS gave me a letter of introduction to the doctor attached to the University of London. I saw him once a month and received my monthly medication from the drug store for one pound under the national health scheme. The medication contained my illness up to January after I had returned from my visit to the continent.

On my return to the residence, which was deserted since most of the students had gone home for the Christmas recess, I started to slide into a depression episode. I started to lose my appetite. I could not get up in the morning, I felt extremely tired most of the time and I felt listless. I felt rejected, I was homesick and I also started feeling hopeless. I lay in my room for days and I could have been committed to hospital or could have become seriously ill if it was not for my friend Jones Mceke. He forced me out of bed, and because the facilities of the residence were not functioning, he saw that I either got to a nearby restaurant or to the cafeteria at Euston station where he virtually forced me to eat something. He washed and ironed my clothing at a nearby launderette and encouraged me to write up my research even if it was only a half-page a day.

My biggest problem was how I was going to cope when the university opened for the new term. I was very scared that if the university authorities discovered that I was depressed they would send me back to South Africa. This had happened to a fellow student from Kenya. I feared imminent disaster because how would I explain my early return from London without completing my studies. This would be a serious let down for the folks at home who had expected so much from me. Thus the battle for survival was on. Jones Mceke accompanied me to the West End where we either watched the latest movies or plays. These and other diversions in London helped to alleviate the depression, but the depression did not lift completely.

God sent me an angel in the form of Jan, a social worker from the PEMHS, who came to London in February 1975 to visit her sister. She visited me and brought me a carton of my favourite cigarettes and took me to the nearest pub round the corner from Euston Station and spent hours on motivating me in a manner that only she could. This did not lift the depression, but made it more manageable. I was still very tired in the mornings and during most of the day, but I dragged myself to meals and forced myself to go on school visits and lectures. My greatest motivation was that although I was depressed, I could not let the fellow blacks down in South Africa.

At about 10 o'clock every night the depression would lift and I would write up my research material even if it were sometimes only a half a page. But I was determined to make a success of my studies. With June approaching we had to complete and hand in our research projects for examination preferably before we left for home, but we were allowed to complete it in our home countries and sent it to the university before the end of a maximum period of 18 months. I was keen to complete my project before I returned home.

Who said God was not with the depression sufferer? With his help and guidance I handed in the three bound copies of my research project to the Chief Advisors of Overseas Students two weeks before I returned to Johannesburg from London.

About 6 months later while at school, I received a large brown envelope which contained a scroll of the University of London. It informed me that I had been awarded the title: "Associate of the Institute of Education of the University of London" for my research project "a Study of the Provision for the Mentally and Physically handicapped in England and Wales and its possible implications for South Africa."

In my humble opinion it was truly a victory for depression sufferers, if I could achieve this little while depressed, what can other fellow depression sufferers not achieve. We as depression sufferers should never give up hope. Do you, the reader, believe in God's miracles? I think my coming through the London experience was a miracle made possible only by a living God.

Having completed my studies at London University I returned to Port Elizabeth to prepare for my marriage on the 16 December 1975.

It was a big struggle to get accommodation in the area which was demarcated for the so called "coloured" population group. I got a temporary room with my sister and her family.

I continued my teaching career at Gelvandale High School which was situated in a Sub economic Township in the Northern Suburbs of Port Elizabeth.

1976 saw the student's protests spilling over to our school. The students refused to attend school and held protest meetings in and around the precinct of the school. They demanded equality of education and herald the slogan "One Man .... One vote."

The security police, by using a system of informers attempted to infiltrate the student body as well as the teaching corps. The police used brutal force and were clearly not prepared to negotiate on any of the student or the broader community's demands.

To me, the behaviour of the police was shocking to what were clearly legitimate demands.

It be soon became apparent that the power of the state would succeed in mollifying the protest, which had taken place all over South Africa

The jest of the parley was the use of Afrikaans as medium of instruction in schools. The majority of black students did not understand the language. 1976 was the turning point of the course of the liberation struggle in South Africa. Since the police had killed many unarmed and protesting students, the African Nationalist Congress (A.N.C.) Pan African Congress (PAC) and National Liberation Front decided to take up arms.

This was the only rational means that the National Party could be overthrown.

With time the situation abated and I returned to the classroom to work under an inferior system of education.

I still had a deep thirst to do educational research.

Mmap Fiction and Drama Series

If you have enjoyed *In the Footsteps of a bipolar life*, consider these other fine books in **Mmap Fiction and Drama Series** from *Mwanaka Media and Publishing*:

The Water Cycle by Andrew Nyongesa
A Conversation…, A Contact by Tendai Rinos Mwanaka
A Dark Energy by Tendai Rinos Mwanaka
Keys in the River: New and Collected Stories by Tendai Rinos Mwanaka
How The Twins Grew Up/Makurire Akaita Mapatya by Milutin Djurickovic and Tendai Rinos Mwanaka
White Man Walking by John Eppel
The Big Noise and Other Noises by Christopher Kudyahakudadirwe
Tiny Human Protection Agency by Megan Landman
Ashes by Ken Weene and Umar O. Abdul
Notes From A Modern Chimurenga: Collected Struggle Stories by Tendai Rinos Mwanaka
Another Chance by Chinweike Ofodile
Pano Chalo/Frawn of the Great by Stephen Mpashi, translated by Austin Kaluba
Kumafulatsi by Wonder Guchu
The Policeman Also Dies and Other Plays by Solomon A. Awuzie
Fragmented Lives by Imali J Abala
In the Beyond by Talent Madhuku
Zororo Risina Zororo by Oscar Gwiriri
Sword of Vengeance by Olatubosun David
Finding A Way Home by Tendai Mwanaka

Your Epistle by Solomon A Awuzie
The Restless Run and Ruin of the Roaches and Rats by McLayode
The Reign of Terror by Ntando Gerald
Ibala Lyabwina Nama by Austin Kaluba
Daddy, Please Don't Kill Mama by Natisha Parsons
Pilate's Angels by Goodenough Mashego
Blue threads and other stories by Matthew Kunashe Chikono

Soon to be released

Conversation with my Mother by Wonder Guchu

https://facebook.com/MwanakaMediaAndPublishing/

www.ingramcontent.com/pod-product-compliance
Lightning Source LLC
Chambersburg PA
CBHW070350270326
41926CB00017B/4078